£15.95 Ins

DICTIONARY
of
NURSING
THEORY
and
RESEARCH

ı2

4

A
DICTIONARY
of
NURSING
THEORY
and
RESEARCH

Second
Edition

Bethel Ann Powers
Thomas R. Knapp

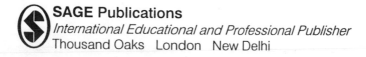
SAGE Publications
International Educational and Professional Publisher
Thousand Oaks   London   New Delhi

For information address:

SAGE Publications, Inc.
2455 Teller Road
Thousand Oaks, CA 91320
E-mail: order@sagepub.com

SAGE Publications Ltd.
6 Bonhill Street
London EC2A 4PU
United Kingdom

SAGE Publications India Pvt. Ltd.
M-32 Market
Greater Kailash I
New Delhi 110 048 India

Printed in the United States of America

Library of Congress Cataloging-in-Publication Data

Powers, Bethel Ann, 1943-
    A dictionary of nursing theory and research / Bethel Ann Powers, Thomas R. Knapp. — 2nd ed.
        p.   cm.
    Includes bibliographical references.
    ISBN 0-8039-5625-8 (cl : alk. paper). — ISBN 0-8039-5626-6 (pb : alk. paper)
    1. Nursing—Research—Dictionaries.   I. Knapp, Thomas R., 1930- II. Title.
    [DNLM: 1. Nursing Theory—dictionaries. 2. Nursing Research—dictionaries.   WY 13 P888d 1995]
    RT81.5.P69   1995
    610.73'03—dc20
    DNLM/DLC   94-46388

This book is printed on acid-free paper.

96 97 98 99 00 01 10 9 8 7 6 5 4 3 2
Sage Project Editor: Susan McElroy

CONTENTS

PREFACE TO THE SECOND EDITION

In this edition of our dictionary all terms presented in the first version have been retained. We have added 66 terms and revised most others. In the process we have also updated our examples and our references.

A word about statistics: Based on reviews of the first edition and conversations with our colleagues and our students, we have added to this edition several statistical terms that are frequently encountered in research reports but were not included in the first edition. Some of those are basic terms such as *mean* and *standard deviation;* they have been briefly defined for the benefit of the beginning researcher. Others are more advanced terms, such as *partial correlation coefficient* and *multicollinearity;* they have been discussed in greater detail and reference has been made to research articles in which those terms are used. But there are many statistical terms that are not included because they are not encountered very often in nursing research reports. Such terms may be found in a number of excellent textbooks in statistics.

We would like to take this opportunity to thank all of you who have given us feedback on the original version and have suggested various ways of making it better. Our special thanks go to Christine Smedley of Sage Publications, to Dr. Jean Brown of the School of Nursing at the State University of New York at Buffalo, to Dr. Julie Buenting of the University of Rochester School of Nursing, and to our students. As always we are grateful for the continued support of our families—Richard and Rachel Powers; Helen, Larry, and Katie Knapp.

Bethel Ann Powers
Thomas R. Knapp

PREFACE TO THE FIRST EDITION

The purpose of *A Dictionary of Nursing Theory and Research* is to provide a handy compilation of definitions and discussions of terms that are commonly encountered in the nursing science literature. Most textbooks in nursing theory or in nursing research contain definitions of terms within the text proper. Some of them also include separate glossaries of those terms. The definitions and glossary entries are usually very brief. As far as we know, there is no source that pulls together the key terms in nursing theory and research, includes extended discussions of those terms, gives examples of situations in which such terms are employed, and provides citations to books and journal articles where the terms are further elaborated. This book is an attempt to fill that void.

Our entries vary considerably in length, with the greatest attention given to those terms that, in our judgment, are the most basic and the most frequently used as well as those terms associated with innovation and change. Cross-references are provided for terms that are often treated in conjunction with one another.

Different textbook authors often define the same term in slightly different ways or use different terms to represent the same thing. We have tried to reflect these matters in our discussions of certain terms. Consider the term *construct*, for example. We try to sort out some of the confusion in the literature regarding the meaning of that term, especially the distinctions that certain authors make between *construct* and *concept*.

This is not the kind of book that you are likely to read from cover to cover. It is a reference source, not a textbook. But if we have been successful in achieving our objective, you will want to keep it very close to your theory and research textbook and/or your collection of professional journals.

This dictionary is intended for undergraduates, graduate students, faculty, and practicing nurses, who may have quite different needs as far as terminology is concerned. The undergraduate nursing student enrolled in an introductory course in research might be interested in something as straightforward as trying to understand the difference between an experiment and a nonexperiment. The advanced doctoral student might care about something as esoteric as the distinctions between two slightly different meanings of the term *multivariate analysis*. Or the reader might want to consider commonalities and differences across different types of qualitative research traditions.

We would like to extend our special thanks to Madeline Schmitt for her careful reading of the entire manuscript and for her very helpful comments and suggestions for improving the exposition. We also thank Jacqueline Fawcett for her encouragement and advice in the early stages of this project. Finally, we thank our families—Richard and Rachel Powers; Helen, Larry, and Katie Knapp—and our students and colleagues over the years who have contributed directly or indirectly to this book through their interest and support.

Bethel Ann Powers
Thomas R. Knapp

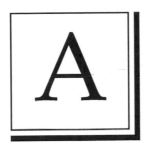

Action Research

Action research is applied research that is oriented toward producing innovation and change. It can be self-evaluative and autobiographical, involving, for example, examination of one's own caring practices or teaching activities; or it can be collaborative, emphasizing the role of participants as partners and stakeholders in studies that are responsive to their interests and concerns.

See **Applied Research**.

Aesthetic Inquiry

Aesthetic knowledge deals with art and perception of meaning through symbolic representations such as fictional narratives, poetry, drawings, paintings, sculpture, music, films, and photographs. Human science researchers regularly use the worlds of art and literature as data sources that stimulate reflection, promote insights, and facilitate writing about lived experience (Munhall, 1994). Sandelowski (1994), in Morse's volume *Critical Issues in Qualitative Research Methods*, discusses art and science as distinct domains that also share a number of continuities:

A

> Art and science are . . . akin to each other in their search for truth, in that they both represent reality, and in the presence of aesthetic criteria governing both domains. . . . In both art and science, we make aesthetic choices, selecting frames of reference and modes of representation for reasons beyond their scientific or artistic merits. . . . Accordingly science cannot claim such things as truth, rigor, or explanation solely for itself; and art cannot claim such things as beauty, imagination, and poetic license solely for itself. Whether we are motivated by impulses to make our work more scientific or artistic, we still make it up. (pp. 51, 54)

Qualitative research is recognized as being "at the crossroads" between art and science, where researchers may choose to "refuse" or "celebrate" aesthetic and artistic possibilities (Sandelowski, 1994). Celebrating the art recognizes the usefulness of nonscientific sources to enhance analysis and permits experimentation with different styles for representing research findings. It does not replace obligations to maintain the rigor and to observe the assumptions, rules, and practices of a particular research tradition. In other words, there is a continuity between art and science that facilitates intellectual tasks and supports different modes of expressiveness in qualitative work. However, there also are distinctions between the two domains that place limits on the ways in which art informs research practice.

From another perspective, some nurse scholars are extending and pursuing the conversation about aesthetic inquiry along the lines of a more "radical reimagining" of the discipline (Chinn & Watson, 1994, p. xvi). Chinn (1994), in Chinn and Watson's anthology *Art and Aesthetics in Nursing*, observes the relationship between art and science to be as follows:

> Art is not something that stands in opposition to science; it is part of science—indeed, it is part of all human experience. Art expresses what words usually fail to express. Art brings wholeness to human consciousness. . . . Art is both feared and revered, because it moves consciousness into realms not imagined and realities not predicted. . . . However, in modern culture, art and science have been ripped apart. (pp. 20-21)

Chinn and Watson's (1994) focus on art and aesthetics seeks to restore "what has been lost" through what they believe to be "denial of the ancient tradition arising from women's healing arts"—a denial, encouraged by the "scientific community," that maintains a false dichotomy between art and science in nursing (p. 21).

Carper's (1978) work on patterns of knowing in nursing provides the conceptual foundation for aesthetic inquiry. Carper (1978) challenged the primacy of empirical research traditions in knowledge development by describing empirics as only one pattern of knowing within a larger whole that includes three other equally important components: personal knowledge, ethics, and aesthetics. Chinn and Kramer (1995), in outlining methods for knowledge development in each of the four areas, observe that personal knowledge and aesthetics are forms of knowing that are best represented symbolically or metaphorically.

Chinn (1994) identifies two types of scholarship that may constitute a methodology for aesthetic inquiry: "(1) critical hermeneutics as applied in the human sciences and (2) art criticism derived from the humanities.... Hermeneutics (defined as the science of interpretation in philosophy) and criticism (defined as the science of resymbolizing in the arts) converge to form a possible new method that can be developed to create new understandings of the art of nursing" (p. 26). The method of aesthetics that she advocates is called aesthetic experiential criticism, an integration of context and meaning in which the evolving research experience and researcher perspectives are subjected to the same degree of analysis as the substantive data (p. 32). Chinn's (1994) example of work in progress with a group of nurse co-researchers involves an examination of the art of nursing practice in three acute care settings, using photographs, vignettes, and personal journaling:

> Critical and creative insights emerge cooperatively within the process of gathering the vignettes or photographs. Discussion then focuses on self-reflective meanings of the situation, and the group explores the many meanings that co-exist, some shared and some not shared. . . . Journaling is primarily self-reflective, but journal entries are brought into experiential process by reading excerpts to other participants as a way of placing before the group possible meanings, metaphors, and symbols that arise from reflection. (p. 33)

The works of Benner (Benner, 1983, 1984; Benner & Tanner, 1987; Benner & Wrubel, 1989) that use a phenomenological hermeneutic approach to explore the art of caring within nursing practice have been credited as contributing to the grounding of methods for aesthetic inquiry. See also (a) Bournaki and Germain's (1993) analysis of aesthetic nursing knowledge in family-centered nursing care of hospitalized children; (b) Schoenhofer's (1994) use of a fictional account about the timeworld of Einstein's dreams to reflect on new visions for the future of nursing; and (c) *Advances in Nursing Science* (1994, volume 17, number 1) issue on "Esthetics and the Art of Nursing." However, scholarly interest in aesthetic patterns of knowing is yet evolving, leaving open further definition of the scope of the field, refinement of methods, and development of a critical mass of work.

See **Art**.

Alternative Hypothesis

An alternative hypothesis is a hypothesis that is pitted against the null hypothesis. It often emerges from theory and is the hypothesis that the investigator usually believes to be true prior to carrying out the research.

An alternative hypothesis is "accepted" when the null hypothesis is rejected, or rejected when the null hypothesis is "accepted." (The word *accepted* is set off in quotation marks because it does not mean that the hypothesis has been proven to be true. It means only that the evidence against it is not sufficiently strong.)

Alternative hypotheses can be specific or nonspecific, and directional (with respect to the null hypothesis) or nondirectional. In contrast, null hypotheses, to be directly testable, must be specific.

Example: The null hypothesis that there is no relationship between age and pulse rate has several alternatives, including (a) there is an inverse relationship of −.50 (specific, directional); (b) the absolute value of the relationship is .50 (specific, nondirectional); (c) there is an inverse relationship (nonspecific, directional); and (d) there is a relationship (nonspecific, nondirectional).

Analysis of Covariance

The analysis of covariance (ANCOVA) is a procedure for testing the significance of the difference among "adjusted" sample means. The means are adjusted to take into account the difference among the corresponding means on an antecedent variable (usually a "pretest" of some sort) and the degree of correlation between that variable and the variable of principal interest. The investigator attempts to determine if the magnitude of the difference among the means is over and above what would be predictable from the antecedent variable.

For an example of the use of analysis of covariance, see Tappen's (1994) report on the effect of skill training on functional abilities of nursing home residents with dementia.

Analysis of Variance

The analysis of variance (ANOVA) is a procedure for testing the significance of the difference among (unadjusted) sample means. "One-way" analysis of variance is used to test the main effect of a single independent variable. Factorial analysis of variance is used to test the main effect of each of two or more independent variables, and their interaction(s). Multivariate analysis of variance (MANOVA) is used when there is more than one dependent variable.

Gulick's (1994) article on social support among persons with multiple sclerosis provides an example of a study in which factorial analysis of variance was used.

Anonymity

Anonymity is associated with the protection of research subjects so that their identities are not known, even to the researcher. This can be accomplished, for example, by the use of an anonymous questionnaire. Anonymity should not be confused with confidentiality, which has to do with not revealing information about subjects, including who they are. In either case the object is to assure that subjects' identities are not linked with their responses.

See **Confidentiality** and **Informed Consent**.

Antecedent Variable

An antecedent variable, A, is a variable that is temporally prior to the independent variable, X, in an $X \rightarrow Y$ causal sequence (where Y is the dependent variable) and could therefore be playing a causal role equal to or greater than that of X itself.

The study of cause-and-effect relationships often includes a search for such variables, that is, precursors of the variable alleged to be the cause (X). This can be especially important in health science research where knowledge of what preceded X could lead to the possibility of control by preventing undesired effects, or by producing or promoting desired effects.

Example: In attempting to determine whether or not stress (X) causes depression (Y), an investigator may discover that it is social support (A)—actually *lack* of social support—that leads to stress, which in turn leads to depression. Therefore social support has an indirect effect on depression "through" stress.

A

Applied Research

Applied research is concerned with using knowledge generated by an investigation to develop practical approaches to problematic situations.

Findings may be less generalizable than those of basic research because of the focus on specific problems. However, there is complementarity between the two approaches when the usefulness of new knowledge produced by basic research is tested by applied research.

See **Research, Basic Research, Action Research, Evaluation Research**, and **Need Analysis**.

Archival Research

Archival research is an activity, integral to various types of investigations, that involves the use of archives. For example, historians and biographers do archival research. Smith (1994) discusses the use of public archives and creation of home study archives in a discussion of biographical method:

> The archival work begins the construction of the life . . . no one library or home study . . . contains all of the papers that are important for the life story. . . . Finding ["pools of data"] is another . . . [aspect of the work]. . . . [However,] the general point is clear: One either finds or builds a data file, an archive, as one step in the process of doing biography. (p. 291)

See Hill (1993) for a discussion of archival strategies and techniques.

Archives

Archives are places where public records or historical documents are preserved. Persons in charge of archives are called archivists.

Government buildings, museums, and libraries typically house archives. Additionally, the storage and rapid retrieval capacities of computers have facilitated an increasing number of database archives in all of the sciences. Individual researchers also may create their own archives, or data files.

Arm

The number of treatments in a randomized clinical trial is occasionally referred to as the number of "arms." The traditional study with one experimental group and one control group has two "arms."

See **Randomized Clinical Trial**.

Armchair Theory

Armchair theory is a term that sometimes is used with reference to theory that has been constructed through cognitive activities, without the use of research methods. Logic, systematic reasoning, and rational argument are used to analyze concepts and describe theoretical relationships.

The negative connotation of armchair theory as a casual compilation of ideas reflects its history in professional jostling between theorists and researchers. However, theory development needs to be a collaborative effort. Both cognitive and research activities are essential in a discipline. Theorists who prefer dealing with the logical connections between abstract ideas complement researcher colleagues who generate, apply, and test theory through scientific investigation.

In her discussion of qualitative secondary analysis, Thorne (1994) pushes the idea of continuities between armchair theorizing and research further by suggesting that armchair induction, in some circumstances, can constitute a form of research:

> Thus secondary analysis creates one rather powerful opportunity for contributions within the qualitative research tradition by those whose aptitudes are more remote from the data source. . . . Armchair induction [is a variety of research] in which those whose talents lie in theory development, rather than engagement with the phenomenon under study, can apply inductive methods of textual analysis, such as hermeneutical inquiry, to existing data sets. (p. 266)

See **Theory** and **Secondary Analysis**.

Art

Art is a particular, subjective expression of aesthetic knowing. "Esthetic knowing in nursing is made visible through the actions, bearing, conduct, attitudes, and interactions of the nurse in response to others" (Chinn & Kramer, 1995, p. 10). Scholarly exploration of aesthetic knowing and art in nursing contributes to theory development in ways that are different from but complementary to empirically focused scientific investigation.

Exploration is grounded in nursing practice. Art expressed through caring nursing actions and performance of skilled tasks has been the focus of research by Benner (Benner, 1984; Benner & Wrubel, 1989). Use of other cultural art forms, such as music, dance, and poetry, to advance understanding is discussed in Chinn and Watson's (1994) anthology *Art and Aesthetics in Nursing.*

See **Aesthetic Inquiry.**

Artifact

In quantitative research, artifact is an artificial result that is not a characteristic of the study phenomenon, but instead is produced by instruments or measurement procedures used in the research. The Hawthorne Effect is an example of artifact, as well as ceiling effect and halo effect in evaluation research. Artifact can be discovered and/or avoided by multiple independent measures or the use of randomly assigned experimental and control groups.

In qualitative research, the possibilities for introducing bias through the methods used by the researcher to collect and analyze data are of equal concern, and various validation and auditing procedures are used to assure accuracy and maintain rigor throughout the investigational process. However, qualitative researchers tend not to use the term *artifact* in connection with these issues.

See **Hawthorne Effect, Ceiling Effect,** and **Halo Effect.**

Artifacts

Artifacts constitute the physical evidence of material culture. They can be anything produced by humans from any point in history, such as written documents, records, and photographs; personal items, such as clothing and jewelry; or products, such as art, tools, and utensils. The study of material culture is of interest in a number of different disciplines in history, the arts, and the social sciences. The research is interpretive in nature.

Hodder (1994) discusses the importance of artifact analysis in understanding social experience, citing such examples as (a) studies of people's garbage that indicated different things about lifestyle and sometimes contradicted subjects' self-reports and (b) studies of "silent discourse conducted by women whose voice has been silenced by dominant male interests," as evidenced by the decoration and arrangement of the household:

> Material traces of behavior give an important and different insight from that provided by any number of questionnaires. "What people say" is often very different from "what people do.". . . The study of material culture is thus of importance for qualitative researchers who wish to explore multiple and conflicting voices, differing and interacting inter-

pretations . . . material culture is not simply a passive by-product of other areas of life. Rather material culture is active. By this I mean that artifacts are produced so as to transform, materially, socially, and ideologically. (pp. 394-395)

In addition to research focused specifically on material culture, attention to artifacts, or the materials that people surround them-selves with in their everyday lives, is a natural aspect of many types of qualitative studies. For example, observation of and discussion about personal artifacts frequently facilitates and enhances data col-lection on topics related to such things as memories, personal experi-ence, lifestyle, and family relationships.

Assay

In nursing "bench" research (basic physiological research), an assay is an experimental procedure for measuring some quantity, for exam-ple, the concentration of cotinine in the urine.

Workman and Livingston (1993) give an example of research that was designed to test the sensitivity (in the precision sense) of an assay for mutagenicity.

Assumption

An assumption is a notion that is taken to be true. Some assump-tions are consistent with particular views of the world and of reality. For example, Lincoln and Guba (1985) contrast traditional science (P = positivist) and qualitative (N = naturalist) assumptions about the nature of reality (ontology) and the relationship of knower to the known (epistemology):

1. The nature of reality
   P—reality is single, tangible, and fragmentable
   N—realities are multiple, constructed, and holistic
2. The relationship of knower to the known
   P—Knower and known are independent, a dualism
   N—Knower and known are interactive, inseparable (p. 37)

Assumptions of this sort are used to support different approaches to theorizing and conducting research. Although they may not be sus-ceptible to being tested empirically, they can be argued philosophi-cally.

A

Other assumptions are made on the basis of tentative support through previous research. For example, in research on patient perceptions of quality of life after coronary artery surgery, King, Porter, Norsen, and Reis (1992) assumed that it would be more beneficial for patients to focus on concrete aspects of their experience than it would be for them to focus attention on the emotional or affective aspects. That assumption was based on a large body of theory and research on coping.

Assumptions may be based on accepted knowledge or personal beliefs and values. They may be identified and stated in the written work of theorists and researchers, but many are not. It then becomes the responsibility of the reader to discover or infer what an author's assumptions may be on the basis of other written statements.

Fawcett (1995) has identified a number of assumptions as part of her evaluations of the conceptual models of nursing by Johnson, King, Levine, Neuman, Orem, Rogers, and Roy. Underlying assumptions are associated with philosophical claims, which need to be made explicit to further understanding of the particular view of nursing that each model represents.

Another type of assumption is associated with methodology. For example, in the "pooled" t test for independent sample means there are the assumptions of normality and homogeneity of variance. Assumptions may also be made about the reliability and validity of study instruments, about the ability of study subjects to understand their roles in the research and to respond appropriately, and about accuracy in data collecting and analysis procedures.

Attenuation

Attenuation is a word that means reduction. In nursing research the term is associated with instrument reliability. The correlation between two measures is occasionally "corrected" for the attenuation that is attributable to any unreliability that might be present in either or both measures.

See **Reliability**.

Attrition

Attrition is the loss of subjects from a study while it is still in progress. In experimental designs, loss of too many subjects can jeopardize the outcome by altering the comparability of the groups. Consequently, in designing the study, determinations of sample size need to take attrition into account.

Audit Trail

In qualitative research, audit trails are created by careful documentation of the research process and sufficient evidence to make it possible for interested others to understand how researchers reached their conclusions. This auditing technique to facilitate validation of research was developed by Halpern (1983) and reported by Lincoln and Guba (1985, pp. 319-320). Six categories of documentation are suggested: (a) raw data—audiotapes, videotapes, field notes, and other documents and records; (b) data reduction and analysis products—write-ups and summaries of field notes and analytic notes; (c) data reconstruction and synthesis products—categories, themes, interpretations, and conclusions; (d) process notes—notes on methods, design, and rigor; (e) materials related to intentions and dispositions—proposal and personal notes; and (f) instrument development information—data collection schedules, interview and observation formats, and surveys.

See Rodgers and Cowles (1993) for further discussion of the types of data that contribute to credible investigations and strategies for record keeping and data management in qualitative research.

Axiom

An axiom is a proposition that is presumed to be true. Axioms are used in the field of mathematics and in formal logical arguments as introductory premises that lead to concluding statements called theorems.

See **Theory**.

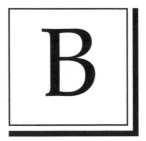

Baseline

A baseline constitutes the measurement of variables or description of a phenomenon prior to implementation of the study conditions, such as intervention, measurement of the effects of other variables, or evaluation of a program or individual performance. For example, in a pretest-posttest approach, the pretest establishes the baseline.

Basic Research

Basic research primarily is concerned with developing the knowledge base and extending theory in academic and/or practice disciplines. In contrast to applied research, findings cannot always be applied directly to practice. However, their abstract, theoretical nature makes them generalizable to a variety of situations, and their utility may be tested through applied research.

See **Research** and **Applied Research**.

Basic Social Process (BSP)

In grounded theory, a basic social process (BSP) is a theoretical summarization of a pattern that people go through in some aspect of their social lives (living with a chronic disease; adjusting to a new situation; coping with loss). Generally, it consists of stages and occurs regardless of the variety of conditions under which it takes place and ways in which people go through it.

See **Grounded Theory**.

Bias

Although used in a variety of contexts in theory and research (Last's, 1988, dictionary of epidemiology contains 27 entries involving the term), *bias* is always associated with some systematic, nonrandom, usually undesirable phenomenon.

Researchers are said to be biased if they are not objective when pursuing their research. A sample is said to be biased if it is not representative of the population about which inferences are to be made. A test is said to be biased if it is unduly difficult for one or more segments of some population. Even a statistic is said to be biased if it systematically underestimates or overestimates some parameter for which it is an estimate.

Techniques for eliminating, controlling, or reducing bias permeate the scientific literature. The use of random samples rather than convenience samples and the random assignment of subjects to treatments in true experiments are just two of the many ways that investigators can control their conscious or unconscious biases. Using test items that are answered correctly by equal percentages of males and females can eliminate sex bias in psychological measurement. Dividing the sum of the squared deviations from the sample mean by one less than the number of observations, rather than the actual number of observations, produces an unbiased estimate of the population variance.

Example: In constructing a test of attitudes toward abortion, one might be advised to select an equal number of statements from "pro-choice" and from "right-to-life" pronouncements as the basis for the test items, to minimize any bias for or against abortion that the investigator might happen to have.

Some controls for bias in data collection and interpretation that qualitative researchers build into the research design are: cross-checking informants' stories, drawing on a variety of data sources, critical self-reflection to account for researchers' own perceptions, systematic data collection, and analysis of possible effects of researchers' actions and involvement in natural settings. Purposeful and theoretical sampling strategies aim to reduce the likelihood of distortion by deliberately varying cases to obtain the broadest possible point of view. An audit trail of careful documentation is another way to control for bias in the research process, by establishing a means for review of the evidence and the decision-making process on which conclusions are based.

Biographical Method

Biographical method is associated with a variety of written representations of people's lives—"portrayals, portraits, profiles, memoirs, life stories, life histories, case studies, autobiographies, journals, diaries, and on and on—each suggesting a slightly different perspective under consideration" (Smith, 1994, p. 287).

With historical roots in literature, history, and the social sciences, biographical method has been effectively used to give voice to feminist and minority perspectives: "Much of recent life writing in professional education carries the same intellectual flavor of the feminist and minority perspective, finding voice among the disenfranchised, the powerless, or those with alternative visions" (Smith, 1994, p. 301).

Nurse historians have used biographical method to examine individuals' achievements and their influence on the discipline. See, for example, Allison (1993), Donahue (1983), Poslusny (1989), Sarnecky (1993), and Widerquist (1992). See also Denzin's (1989) discussion of biographical method.

Blocking

Blocking is a combination of matching and random assignment used in the design of experiments. The experimenter first creates a set of matched pairs with respect to some variable of interest (for example, intelligence or income) and then randomly assigns one member of each pair to the experimental group and the other member to the control group.

Blocking is to the sample as stratifying is to the population. One blocks the sample to control for a possibly confounding variable; one stratifies the population before sampling so that the sample will be representative of the population with respect to that variable.

See **Control**.

Blurred Genres

The idea of blurred genres was advanced by Clifford Geertz in two works, *The Interpretation of Cultures* (1973) and *Local Knowledge* (1983), in which he proposed that the boundaries between the social sciences and the humanities had become blurred. That is, he observed that new approaches were emerging across disciplines, particularly as social

14

scientists expressed greater interest in and began to use theories, methods, and representational styles from the humanities.

References in the literature to "blurring" of distinctions across disciplines or between various traditions of theory and research derive from this notion.

Borrowed Theory

A borrowed theory is theory developed in another discipline that is not adapted to the worldview and practice of nursing. "There is, however, increasing awareness of the need to test borrowed theories to determine if they are empirically adequate in nursing situations" (Fawcett, 1995, p. 26).

The term *borrowed theory* has a history in earlier theory debates about the need for unique theory in nursing. It is not consistent with the view that knowledge belongs to the scientific community and to society at large, and is not the property of individuals or disciplines.
See **Theory**

Bracketing

Bracketing, in phenomenology and other qualitative traditions, involves identifying and holding suspended previously acquired knowledge, beliefs, and opinions about a phenomenon under study. The term *bracketing* was borrowed from mathematics by Edmund Husserl (1859-1938), himself a mathematician as well as the "father of phenomenology" (van Manen, 1990, pp. 175-176).

See **Phenomenology**.

Broad-Range Theory

Broad-range theory deals with wide areas of concern in a discipline, covering a number of phenomena that relate to larger wholes, for example, a conceptualization of nursing's goal for health promotion and maintenance for all individuals in a society. Other labels that reflect a theory that is broad in scope and deals with multiple phenomena and patterns that make up a larger whole include macrotheory, holistic theory, and grand theory.

"Examples of broad-range or grand theories in nursing include Leininger's (1991) theory of culture care diversity and universality, Newman's (1986) theory of health as expanding consciousness, and Parse's (1981, 1992) theory of human becoming" (Fawcett, 1995, p. 25).

See **Theory**.

B

Buffering Variable

A buffering variable, B, is a type of intervening variable that mediates (beneficially) the effect of an independent variable, X, on a dependent variable, Y.

Example: In some theories regarding the effect of stress (X) on depression (Y), social support (B) is said to play a buffering rather than an antecedent role in that the effect of stress is lessened in proportion to the extent of positive social support available to an individual (large network size, density, reciprocity, etc.). This hypothesis is an integral element in the work of Norbeck (1981) and others. Evidence for the stress-buffering effect of social support has been summarized by Thoits (1982), and some methodological considerations regarding the testing of buffering effects of social support and coping are discussed by Finney, Mitchell, Cronkhite, and Moos (1984).

See **Antecedent Variable, Intervening Variable,** and **Mediating Variable.**

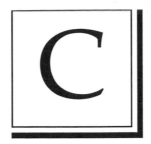

Canonical Correlation Analysis

Canonical correlation analysis is a type of multivariate analysis concerned with the relationships between linear composites of two sets of variables. One set typically consists of one or more independent variables and the other set typically consists of one or more dependent variables, but the independent versus dependent distinction is sometimes not relevant.

It can be shown that canonical correlation analysis subsumes multiple regression analysis, the analysis of variance, and several other traditional analyses.

Wikoff and Miller (1991) give an example of the use of canonical correlation analysis in a longitudinal study of myocardial infarctions.

See **Multivariate Analysis**.

Case-Control Study

A case-control study is a retrospective epidemiological study in which subjects who have contracted a particular disease (the "cases") are compared with similar subjects who did not contract the disease (the "controls"). The term *disease* is often used quite liberally to include such things as having an abortion or failure to follow a prescribed regimen of medication.

The article by Polivka and Nickel (1992) discusses the applicability of case-control studies to nursing research and provides an example of such a study.

See **Epidemiological Research**.

Case Study

A case study is an intensive in-depth investigation of a single subject or a single unit, which could be a small number of individuals who seem to be representative of a larger group or very different from it. Families, organizations, institutions (colleges, factories, hospitals), programs, and events also could be the unit of analysis. Some research situations call for a multiple or comparative case study approach. (See Schultz & Kerr, 1986, for an example of comparative case study research in community health.) Case studies have been used to good advantage in other disciplines. Hypotheses derived from ideas generated from Freud's case studies of clients with personality disorders continue to be tested and systematically studied into the present. The fields of law and ethics rely on case analysis. Anthropologists frequently use a case study approach in analyzing a community and individuals who are thought to be either typical or atypical members of it.

Research questions that lend themselves to the case study approach are usually less concerned with measuring the effects of isolated variables on one another and more concerned with discovering what the relevant variables are that may explain, for example, why a study subject thinks and acts in certain ways, how a program was implemented, or how and why a particular event took place. (Case studies deal with contemporary events in contrast to historical studies, which tend to focus on past events.) Yin (1989) differentiates among descriptive (looking at a case from different angles), exploratory (debating the value of further investigating various hypotheses or propositions), and explanatory (examining various aspects of a causal argument) case studies.

Some case studies involve the administration of a treatment or intervention and the description of its effects. Holm (1983) asserts that the "experimental approach" taken in single-subject research is a modification of experimental design principles. This includes recording baseline measures of the dependent variable, introducing the treatment/intervention, subsequent recording of the dependent variable, and comparing findings from baseline and treatment/intervention phases.

C

In case study design, the researcher selects and combines data-gathering approaches that are most relevant to the study. Multiple data sources are used, such as records and documents, questionnaires and interviews, direct observation, participant observation, rating scales, physiological or psychological measures, and physical artifacts (products of culture—art and technology). Case studies may involve extensive documentation of subjects' responses in nonexperimental and natural environments over a substantial period of time. The investigator may explore people's past histories to gain insights about, and generate interpretations of, their current thoughts and actions. However, case studies need not include detailed observation and interview data as sources of evidence. The analysis can be limited to various forms of quantitative data. Also, case study research should not be confused with qualitative research. Not every case study incorporates a qualitative perspective, and qualitative investigations can but do not always produce case studies (Yin, 1989).

Analysis of results is of two types. Idiographic analysis concerns itself with particulars—the unique aspects of persons, events, or things. Generalizations are restricted to the specific case. For example, predictions about future behavior may be made on the basis of interpretations of past behavior. Nomothetic analysis is focused on finding general laws that subsume individual cases. It involves generalizing from one case to a larger group of which it is thought to be representative or comparing the single case with another known group to identify differences. Some researchers argue that important features of one case may little resemble what is to be found in another, and therefore generalization across cases cannot be supported. Others argue that if it can be established that one person responds to or experiences things in particular ways, it is reasonable to presume that others could react similarly. One side of the argument focuses on probabilities and the other on possibilities. Lincoln and Guba (1985) describe the nomothetic-idiographic "dilemma" as one that particularly "haunts" the helping professions where professionals try to deal with an individual's problems by using general principles or theories, which then must be examined to see if they apply to the unique case. Lincoln and Guba (1985) suggest that perhaps case law is the best example of successfully dealing with the problem because it is "built largely on precedent cases . . . that are powerful precisely because they take particulars into account" (p. 117).

For examples of case studies, such as the one by Wells, Williamson, and Hooker (1994) about an 8-year-old girl who had undergone repair

19

of coarctation of the aorta, see almost any issue of *Maternal-Child Nursing Journal* or *Heart and Lung.*

Categories

In qualitative research, categories are abstract labels that group similar phenomena observed in data. As data are compared for similarities and differences, they are coded. Codes are compared and clustered to form categories of information. Defining, developing, and integrating categories is a major task in some kinds of qualitative research.

The term is also used by quantitative researchers as synonymous with "levels" to indicate the various possible values that a variable can take on.

See **Qualitative Research** and **Variable**.

Causal-Comparative Study

A causal-comparative study is a type of correlational research in which two or more groups are compared with one another, either prospectively or retrospectively, to generate hypotheses regarding relationships between nonexperimental variables.

Studies concerned with the relationship between cigarette smoking and lung cancer are prototypical examples of causal-comparative studies, and most of them are of the retrospective variety.

See **Correlational Research.**

Causality

Causality (sometimes called causation) is a concept associated with the determination of cause-and-effect relationships between variables. Most authors (e.g., Williamson, Karp, Dalphin, & Gray, 1982) list three conditions for establishing that X is *a cause* of Y (there are additional requirements for demonstrating that X is *the cause* of Y—see Last, 1988, for the distinctions regarding necessary vs. sufficient causality):

1. X must precede Y temporally.
2. There must be a strong relationship between X and Y.
3. If $U, V, W, \ldots$ are controlled, the relationship between X and Y still holds, i.e., it is not a spurious relationship.

The claim of a cause-and-effect relationship is usually an outcome of hypothesis testing associated with experimental research. However, attribution of causality is not necessarily limited by type of research design. Testable hypotheses may be derived from findings resulting from nonexperimental research, and there is no research approach that can actually prove causality. It is also important to appreciate that single examples of research are inadequate to support a suggested causal relationship. Consistent replication of research findings is an important determinant of the seriousness with which claims of causality should be taken.

Example: It is alleged that cigarette smoking (X) causes lung cancer (Y). The first of the three conditions for causality is taken to be satisfied, as it is most unlikely that having lung cancer precedes the smoking of cigarettes. The second condition is also satisfied, as hundreds of scientific studies have established that cigarette smoking and lung cancer are closely associated with one another. Except for some highly controlled animal experiments, however, the third condition remains unsatisfied, as smoking/cancer studies of human beings have not provided sufficient controls to rule out other confounding factors such as air pollution (U) or genetic disposition (V) as cancer-causing factors, rather than cigarette smoking itself.

Ceiling Effect

Ceiling effect is the phenomenon whereby judges or evaluators score almost everyone, as the term implies, at or near the top of a scale. This makes it impossible to rank-order performance and creates little opportunity for major individual improvement with subsequent performances.

Ceiling effect may be addressed by revisiting instructions for scoring performance and by evaluating the way in which the judges perform the evaluations.

See **Artifact**.

Cell

A cell is a portion of a cross-tabulation that contains the frequency associated with a category of one variable in combination with a category of another variable.

See **Cross-Tabulation**.

Chi-Square Test

A chi-square test is a test of statistical significance usually carried out on cross-tabulated data that summarize the relationship between two nominal variables.

In their study of complications associated with prenatal genetic procedures, Stringer and Librizzi (1994) use the chi-square test.

See **Cross-Tabulation** and **Test of Significance**.

Cluster Sampling

Cluster sampling is a type of multistage sampling for which the initial stage consists of the selection of groups of subjects rather than individual subjects.

See **Sampling**.

Coding

Coding is a process of breaking down raw research data into some form in which they can be manipulated, organized, and examined more easily. Coding may involve assigning numerical symbols to bits of data so that they can be computerized. Codes may also consist of word labels and phrases that attempt to capture or stand for some central idea that qualitative data convey to the researcher.

See **Dummy Variable** and **Qualitative Research**.

Coefficient Alpha (Cronbach's Alpha)

Coefficient alpha, also known as Cronbach's alpha (the educational psychologist, Lee J. Cronbach, 1951, derived it), is an index of the degree to which a measuring instrument is internally reliable. It indicates how well the items correlate with one another, as the following formula for *standardized* alpha shows:

$$\text{alpha} = \frac{k\bar{r}}{1 + (k-1)\bar{r}}$$

where k is the number of items and $\bar{r}$ is the average correlation between pairs of items

Coefficient alpha is the average of all possible "split-half" reliabilities for a k-item instrument. Although it is the most commonly reported indicator of the reliability of an instrument, coefficient alpha is subject to a number of problems. See the article by Knapp (1991) for details.

Example: A 26-item test of nursing aptitude for which the average inter-item correlation is .20 would have a standardized coefficient alpha of $26(.20)/[1 + 25(.20)] = .87$.

A note of caution: This statistic has nothing at all to do with Type I error or with the intercept for a population regression equation. Unfortunately all three are called "alpha."

See **Reliability**.

Cohort

A cohort is a group of people who share some demographic event, usually birth. In longitudinal studies one or more cohorts of research subjects are followed across time in order to investigate age-related changes.

The term *cohort effect* is used to refer to the phenomenon whereby a result obtained for a particular cohort may be limited to that cohort and not generalizable.

Example: One of the most interesting and most frequently studied cohorts is "the baby boom cohort," which consists of the generation of people born right after World War II, more specifically the birth years from 1946 through 1964.

Computer-Assisted Research

The possibilities for use of computer-assisted methods in research are numerous and expanding, with ongoing developments in computer technology and software design. Packages that perform statistical computations have long been available, and, more recently, there has been an explosion of computer software for the management and analysis of narrative text.

A computer package is a collection of computer programs that carry out a variety of statistical analyses. Some computer packages are very expensive and require a special site license. Most are available for both mainframes and PCs. The best-known computer packages are the Statistical Analysis System (SAS) and the Statistical Package for the Social Sciences (SPSS). Others that are occasionally mentioned in research reports are BMDP, MINITAB (very popular with statisticians for the teaching of statistics), SYSTAT, and SYSTAT's "miniversion" MYSTAT (which is available free of charge for the asking or with the purchase of statistics texts such as Munro & Page, 1993).

Software programs for qualitative researchers provide assistance with descriptive/interpretive and theory-building tasks. Programs for descriptive/interpretive functions permit the user to attach codes to segments of text and will then at the user's instruction rapidly retrieve and assemble all of the segments that were coded in a certain way. In addition to these two main functions, enhanced programs perform various special functions, such as searching for multiple codes, searching for a particular sequence of codes, or counting the frequency of the occurrence of codes. Programs designed to support theory building permit development of an indexing or organizing system that can be added to and modified as the researcher thinks about potential relationships within the data.

While computer-assisted methods streamline data management, it is important to remember that the machine does *not* analyze data. Researchers analyze data. If incorrect data are entered, if the coding is sloppy, or if the logic is faulty, the computer will not "know." The computer only follows instructions.

Of equal importance is the need for researchers to remain true to the intellectual commitments of the particular mode in which they are working. The computer is the servant, not the master—that is, the analytic procedures should not be tailored to the capacities of the program. Instead, the researcher may have to spend some time and effort looking for the program that will fit the specific needs of the analysis. The proliferation of programs attests to this type of experience, where researchers have worked with computer programmers to develop new computer applications.

Finally, qualitative researchers, in particular, find that computerization has both advantages and limitations:

> Artificial intelligence research has thus contributed to qualitative analysis powerful techniques for managing not only documents but also concepts, and for constructing and expressing theories. Many researchers may of course never want these features, and will use computers for enhanced code-and-retrieve for collecting related passages for their contemplation . . . although software designs imported from artificial intelligence and database research are providing the breakthroughs, none of them is exactly what QDA [qualitative data analysis] needs. The problem and the excitement is that QDA is probably the most subtle and intuitive of human epistemological enterprises, and therefore likely to be the last to achieve satisfactory computerization. (Richards & Richards, 1994, pp. 460-461)

For useful discussions of computer-assisted options available to qualitative researchers, see Fielding & Lee (1991); Richards & Richards (1991, 1994); Tesch (1990); and Walker (1993).

See **Informatics**.

Concept

A concept is an idea or complex mental image of a phenomenon (object, property, or event). Concepts are the major components of theory.

See **Theory**.

Concept Analysis

Concept analysis is the systematic examination of the definitions, properties, and attributes of concepts such as Davis's (1992) analysis of pain management or Müller and Dzurec's (1993) analysis of maternal-fetal attachment.

Conceptual Framework

See **Conceptual Model** and **Model**.

Conceptual Model/Conceptual Framework

A conceptual model is a set of interrelated concepts that symbolically represent and convey a mental image of a phenomenon. Conceptual models of nursing identify concepts and describe their relationships to the phenomena of central concern to the discipline: person, environment, health, and nursing.

See **Model**.

Concurrent Validity

Concurrent validity is a type of criterion-related validity in which the data for the predictor and the data for the criterion are collected at essentially the same point in time.

See **Validity**.

Confidence Interval

A confidence interval is a range of values that has some specified probability (usually .95 or .99) of including a particular population parameter.

See **Inferential Statistics** and **Interval Estimation**.

Confidentiality

Confidentiality is associated with the protection of research subjects so that their identities are not revealed or linked with their responses in any way. Confidentiality should not be confused with anonymity, which also has to do with protecting subjects' identities. However, ensuring anonymity requires that even the researcher cannot link respondents' identities to their responses.

See **Anonymity** and **Informed Consent**.

Confounding

Confounding occurs when the effects of two or more independent variables on the dependent variable are entangled with one another (whether or not each of those variables is explicitly part of the study design). It is usually undesirable and occasionally unavoidable.

If it cannot be determined whether it was Variable *A* or Variable *B* that had an effect, but only some hopelessly intermingled combination of the two, the results of the research are extremely difficult to interpret. But confounding is very hard to eliminate, even in well-controlled experiments, because certain treatments come as package deals, so to speak. If Drug A is a pill and Drug B is a liquid, it would be impossible to disassociate the effect of the ingredient from the effect of the form in which the ingredient is delivered.

There are situations, however, in which confounding is deliberately built into the design of the study. When investigating the effects of several independent variables simultaneously, a researcher might intentionally confound two of them, for example, time of day and room location, because there are just too many combinations to test separately or because it is felt unnecessary to isolate the separate effects.

Example: One of the very worst things that could be done when designing a two-treatment, both-sexes study is to assign all of the males to Treatment 1 and all of the females to Treatment 2. If those who received Treatment 1 outperformed those who received Treatment 2, the researcher wouldn't know whether it was a treatment difference or a sex difference (or some combination of the two). The appropriate way to design such a study would be to *randomly* assign *half* of the males to Treatment 1 and the other half to Treatment 2, and to randomly assign half of the females to Treatment 1 and the other half to Treatment 2. This "blocking on sex" would produce *four* groups rather than two, and the main effect of sex, the main effect of treatment, and the sex-by-treatment interaction could all be tested.

Constant Comparative Method

The constant comparative method is a systematic approach to data analysis described by grounded theorists and used by other qualitative researchers. It is part of a search for patterns in data as they are coded, sorted into categories, and examined within different contexts. It involves continuously comparing bits of data as they are separated out, defining the particular characteristics of categories of data, and clarifying relationships between categories.

See **Grounded Theory**.

Construct

A construct is a theoretical dimension that has been or potentially could be operationalized by one or more variables.

The terms *concept* and *construct* are often used interchangeably, but some authors make certain distinctions between the two terms. *Concept* is usually regarded as the more general of the terms. In that case all constructs are concepts, but all concepts are not constructs. *Pain*, for example, is a construct that is also a concept. But *ideal mother* would be regarded by many researchers as a concept but not a construct.

Other authors take the opposite viewpoint regarding the distinction between the two terms. Chinn and Kramer (1995), for example, describe constructs as "the most complex type of concept on the empiric-abstract continuum . . . [including] ideas with a reality base so abstract that it is *constructed* from multiple sources of direct and indirect evidence" (p. 60). Kaplan (1964) classifies concepts on the basis of the extent to which they are observable. His third level is the construct. The first two are the directly observable concept and the indirectly observable concept, and the fourth (and most abstract) level is the theoretical term.

An additional distinction between *construct* (theoretical) and *variable* (operational) is usually necessary. "Intelligence," for example, is a construct whereas "score on the Wechsler Adult Intelligence Scale" is a variable.

In most studies the investigator starts with a construct (which often is an essential component of some theory) and ends up with one or more variables that are alleged to be measures of that construct. But there are also studies that start with the variables and extract the construct. The latter is the approach taken in factor analysis.

The term *construct* is often used in conjunction with *validity*. Construct validity is the kind of validity that is of most interest in theory generation and theory testing.

Example: Obesity is a construct (it is also a concept). An investigator might theorize about obesity and define it in operational terms such as the thickness of certain skin folds, percent of body fat, weight as a percent of average weight for height, and so forth. Alternatively, an investigator might perform a factor analysis and have obesity emerge as a "principal component" of those variables.

See **Concept** and **Variable**.

C

Construct Validity

Construct validity is a type of validity in which the conformity to theoretical expectations of relationships between a previously un- tested measure and other variables is explored.

See **Validity**.

Contamination

Contamination is the term used to refer to a weakness of any experiment in which the treatment groups are not kept sufficiently isolated, so that the subjects who are supposed to receive just one of the treatments actually are exposed to part or all of one of the other treatments.

Example: A researcher in nursing education carries out an experi- ment in a college of nursing in which a random half of student nurses are taught how to give injections using Method A and the other half are taught how to give those same injections using Method B. Since the students attend the same college they have the opportunity to communicate with one another regarding their training, and it is very difficult, if not impossible, for those who are receiving Method A to be completely deprived of the techniques involved in Method B; the experiment is therefore "contaminated."

Content Analysis

Content analysis is a method of managing narrative material and, thus, it has been associated with coding and classifying processes used in some types of qualitative research. This is problematic, be- cause standard texts on the topic (Holsti, 1969; Krippendorff, 1980; Rosengren, 1981) have a more consistent fit with quantitative ("de- ductive-verificatory-enumerative-objective") approaches (Lincoln & Guba, 1985, p. 339). The term alone, then, is not a sufficient descriptor of the analytic methods that will be applied to a particular research project. The researcher will need to be more specific.

The conventional method involves quantification of the content of communications according to predetermined categories. The catego- ries are created on the basis of issues or data characteristics of interest to the researcher; and rules for coding and classifying content as belonging to one or another category are stated precisely, to minimize bias resulting from judgments of different coders. Data reduced to numerical form can then be processed by computers and analyzed statistically. Criticism of the method suggests that creating quantifi- able data from narrative accounts does not enhance their validity or their meaningfulness. Manning and Cullum-Swan (1994) observe that "content analysis has been unable to capture the context within which a written text has meaning" (p. 464).

The method of coding and classifying narrative data in qualitative research can resemble conventional descriptions of content analysis to the extent that qualitative researchers sometimes use the term in connection with their own analytic procedures. However, there are important differences. Qualitative researchers seldom use quantification as described above and do not predetermine the categories into which data will be placed. Rules and procedures are not wholly fixed before the simultaneous data collection/data analysis process begins. Guidelines and rationales for categorizing qualitative research data develop as the analysis unfolds. The concern with bias, objectivity, and replicability that accompanies use of coders trained to manage data according to the established rules is not consistent with a qualitative perspective. And use of content analysts' published schemes for classifying data is an instrumental approach that contrasts with the inductive methods used in qualitative research.

Because the concept of content analysis means different things to researchers, depending upon whether their orientation is primarily quantitative or qualitative, it is always necessary to carefully articulate the actual procedures to be used and to give thought to the assumptions about research that guide their use. The assumptions are important when it comes to consistency of procedures with the chosen approach.

See **Ethnography, Grounded Theory, Qualitative Research,** and **Quantitative Research.**

Content Validity

Content validity is a type of validity in which expert judgment is brought to bear in determining the extent to which a particular variable properly operationalizes some construct of interest.

See **Validity.**

Contingency Table

See **Cross-Tabulation.**

Control

Control is a term that has to do with the assessment of causality. Whenever one is seriously interested in the causal relationship between two variables, whether in a true experiment or in a theoretically oriented correlational study, one must account for extraneous variables that might otherwise render any sort of causal interpretation unjustifiable.

There is a wide variety of procedures for accomplishing such control, but they are all of either a *direct* or a *statistical* nature. The simplest form of direct control of a variable is to hold it constant, for example, to control for sex differences by using only males, or only females, in a particular study. This option is often unwise, however, as it restricts the generalizability of the research findings. Other direct methods include "blocking" on a variable (matching coupled with random assignment to treatment groups) and random assignment alone.

Techniques providing statistical control are the use of change scores, the analysis of covariance, and a variety of other regression methods. Statistical control is always inferior to direct control, as the interpretation must involve the notion "*if* _____ were to be held constant" rather than "*when* _____ is held constant," but it is the only alternative when direct control is either difficult or impossible, for example, in virtually all nonexperimental studies.

Example: An experimental study of the effectiveness of a new drug relative to an old drug would ordinarily employ direct control with some variables held constant at the sampling stage and others "randomized out" in the assignment-to-treatment stage, with or without blocking on something like sex. The "experimental group" would get the new drug and the "control group" would get the old drug; at the end of the study the two groups would be compared on the dependent variable(s) of interest, for example, morbidity or mortality. But a nonexperimental study of the relationship between type of drug and morbidity for people who just happened to have been exposed to various drugs would have to rely entirely on statistical control.

Control Group

In an experiment the control group is the group that does not receive the "treatment" (e.g., a new analgesic) that is of particular interest to the researcher. (It must receive *some* kind of treatment, however—e.g., the usual analgesic—since there is no such thing as a "pure" control group.)

See **Experiment**.

Convenience Sampling

Convenience sampling is the very common type of nonprobability sampling in which the researcher selects any or all available subjects who agree to participate in the study.

Example: College students enrolled in psychology courses provide convenience samples for much of psychological research.

See **Sampling**.

Convergent Validity

Convergent validity is a type of construct validity. If there is a strong relationship between a particular measure and one or more other alleged measures of the same construct, the given measure is said to possess convergent validity.

See **Validity**.

Correlation Coefficient

A correlation coefficient is a number that summarizes the direction and strength of the relationship between two variables. The most commonly encountered correlation coefficient is the Pearson product-moment correlation coefficient.

See **Pearson Product-Moment Correlation Coefficient**.

Correlational Research

Correlational research examines the relationships between variables, but unlike experimental or quasi-experimental studies, correlational studies lack active manipulation of the independent variable(s). Therefore, postulation of relationships among study variables in causal terms is risky. Discussion of associations in correlational studies, however, sometimes gives an indication of how likely it is that a cause-and-effect relationship *might* exist.

Questions such as "Does obesity contribute to the incidence of coronary heart disease?" or "Does a person's cultural background affect perception of and response to pain?" are examples where the independent variable is a characteristic of an individual that cannot be manipulated experimentally. Other questions about the effects of various treatments on people often cannot be studied experimentally because of ethical considerations that would be involved in randomly withholding the treatment of particular interest from some clients. There are also instances where random assignment of subjects to experimental and control groups is impractical or beyond the investigator's ability to carry out.

31

Other advantages cited in the research literature have to do with the capacity of correlational designs to deal with large amounts of data connected with a specific problem area and their strong link to reality in contrast with the artificiality of laboratory experiments.

There are many kinds of correlational research. The most common kind is "ordinary" correlational research in which the interrelationships of pairs of variables are explored. Causal-comparative studies (either prospective or retrospective) compare two or more groups of subjects on one or more variables to determine whether or not there is a "case" for causality.

Example: An investigator's report of a strong relationship between type of nursing care and patient satisfaction may suggest that assignment of patients to a primary nurse is likely to result in greater satisfaction with nursing care.

The following diagram may be helpful in clarifying the various types of correlational research:

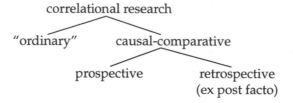

Criterion (Criteria pl.)

A criterion is an external standard against which an object (e.g., performance, a report, a research study) may be judged. Evaluative criteria are derived from agreed-upon norms and expectations that are systematically applied to judge or assess the adequacy of something.

Criterion-related Validity

Criterion-related validity is a type of validity concerned with the relationship between a particular measure and some external "gold standard," that is, a measure whose validity has been assumed or previously demonstrated.

See **Validity**.

Critical Ethnography

Critical ethnography combines an ethnographic research approach with critical inquiry. The result, as described by Thomas (1993), is "conventional ethnography with a political purpose" (p. 4). Street (1992), in *Inside Nursing: A Critical Ethnography of Clinical Nursing Practice*, describes the research process as "openly ideological in design and emancipatory in intent" (p. 8): "An ethnography framed within this context of critical inquiry, predisposed to rationally analyze and change unjust and irrational social activity, was classed as a critical ethnography in order to distinguish it from ethnographies with no transformative agenda whose purpose is framed to describe and interpret cultural realities" (p. 12).

See also Muecke's (1994) discussion of varieties of anthropological ethnographies.

See **Ethnography**, **Critical Social Science**, and **Critical Theory**.

Critical Social Science

Fay (1987) proposes that the term *critical social science* be used to differentiate between the two meanings of critical theory: (a) neo-Marxist theory/a theory of society and (b) a metatheory of science:

> It is important to see that these two senses are different: one can without contradiction subscribe to critical theory understood as a theory of the nature of social science and at the same time believe that the critical theory of modern society given by Habermas et al. is false. . . . In the broadest terms, critical social science is an attempt to understand in a rationally responsible manner the oppressive features of a society such that this understanding stimulates its audience to transform their society and thereby liberate themselves. (pp. 4-5)

See **Critical Ethnography** and **Critical Theory**.

Critical Theory

Critical theory refers to (a) a neo-Marxist theory of society, a theory of advanced capitalism associated with certain members of the Institute of Social Research established in Frankfurt, Germany, in 1923 by Max Horkheimer, Friedrich Pollock, Theodor Adorno, Herbert Marcuse, and Leo Lowenthal (often referred to as the Frankfurt school) and later advanced by Jurgen Habermas *and* (b) a metatheory of science, that is, an extension and development of a form of social analysis and critique.

C

The historical emphasis of critical theory has been on ideology, that is, idea systems produced by the socially elite that tend to be false and to conceal the truth. This orientation toward identifying and critiquing forms of domination was initially stimulated by fascism in the 1930s and 1940s, but it has shifted over time to concerns about domination in modern capitalist societies. A contribution of the critical school of thought been its effort to reorient Marxist theory beyond its strong emphasis on materialism and economic structures toward a broader interest in culture and the subjective concerns of individuals.

Interest in the dialectic has provided another focus. A dialectical process of reasoning involves polar opposites (thesis and antithesis) that in real life could be any set of relationships that are viewed as interactive (e.g., nurse-patient; health-illness). Through examination of the contradictory aspects of their abstract natures, where notions about them clash and collide, a new and more advanced understanding is created (synthesis), which brings growth and fresh outlooks out of the crisis of opposition. The notion of polar opposites is associated with Hegelian-Marxist philosophy and is viewed within critical theory as part of a general law of development that applies equally to nature and society in the real world. That law states that development (change or progress) occurs in dialectical sequences of contradiction and synthesis that can be understood by means of dialectical logic and analysis. Dialogical and dialectical methodology in theory building and research is consistent with the emphasis of critical theory on (a) understanding the world through a grasp of how history affects social circumstances and related ideologies, and (b) generating critical knowledge that raises human self-consciousness to the point of a social movement, resulting in some form of emancipation from oppressive social arrangements or false ideas. The role of criticism (critique) in critical theory has been linked with negative judgments of conventional social norms and dominant ideology. However, the positive contribution is in terms of discovering and unmasking oppressive forms of belief to promote emancipation of people in society. Basic assumptions of this type of analysis are that humans are typically dominated by social conditions that they can neither understand nor control, that human existence does not need to be this way, and that enlightenment about the ideologies that oppress and constrain people can free and empower them. Enlightenment, empowerment, and emancipation are the major concepts. Enlightenment ultimately is knowledge of self in relation to the world and education of the oppressed in terms of their potential capacity to bring about revolutionary change. Empowerment involves social transformation through some form of educative process. Emancipation is a state of broadened rationality and reflective clarity where people have a sense of themselves and can freely and collectively determine the directions they should take in life. Thus, critical theory as an analytic style constitutes a philosophical approach to scientific understanding of society that emphasizes the power of reason to transform people's lives.

Use of critical approaches to analyze social phenomena has spread to many fields. This proliferation of a number of criticalist traditions has given rise to differences beyond their common roots in the theoretical tradition of the Frankfurt school. "Critical theory should not be treated as a universal grammar of revolutionary thought objectified and reduced to discrete formulaic pronouncements or strategies . . . any attempts to delineate critical theory as discrete schools of analysis will fail to capture the hybridity endemic to contemporary criticalist analysis" (Kincheloe & McLaren, 1994, pp. 139, 140).

Theoretical and investigative work in applied disciplines draw on critical theory forms of analyses to advance understanding of diverse practical issues. In the field of education, critical studies have addressed production and reproduction of social class structure through schooling under capitalism. Feminist theory in the area of women's studies addresses issues of sexism in various social situations from a critical perspective. Critical social theory also has been described and promoted as a relevant framework for theory development in nursing, both theoretical and data based.

For additional information about critical theory see Fay (1987), Habermas (1971), and Held (1980). For examples of critical studies see Gilligan (1982), MacLeod (1987), Melosh (1982), and Weiler (1988). For further readings in the nursing literature on critical theory, feminist theory, and the dialectic, see Allen (1985, 1986); Allen, Allman, and Powers (1991); Allen, Benner, and Diekelmann (1986); Allen and Whatley (1986); Campbell and Bunting (1991); Hedin (1986); MacPherson (1983); McLain (1988); Moccia (1985, 1986); Stevens (1989); Wild (1993); and Wilson and Fitzpatrick (1984).

See **Critical Ethnography, Critical Social Science, Dialectic, Dialogical Inquiry, Discourse Analysis,** and **Feminist Methodology.**

Cronbach's Alpha
See **Coefficient Alpha.**

Crossover Design

A crossover design, sometimes called a counterbalanced design, is an experimental design in which every subject is exposed to both of two experimental treatments in a balanced fashion. At Time 1 half of the subjects receive Treatment A and the other half receive Treatment B. At Time 2 they "cross over," with the first half receiving Treatment B and the second half receiving Treatment A.

Crossover designs are special cases of "Latin square" designs in which each of k treatments is administered to each of k groups of subjects at k points in time (where k is equal to or greater than 2).

Whitney, Stotts, Goodson, and Janson-Bjerklie (1993) used a crossover design in their study of effects of activity and bed rest on tissue oxygen tension, perfusion, and plasma volume.

Cross-Sectional Study

The term *cross-sectional study* is sometimes used in a general sense to classify any study that does not involve a follow-up of the research subjects. For example, a study in which one group of subjects is recruited over a relatively long period of time but is never followed up thereafter, could be labeled a cross-sectional study. In its more restrictive technical sense, however, a cross-sectional study is a type of study that involves the comparison of two or more groups (e.g., age groups) at one point in time, as opposed to a longitudinal study that traces a cohort of people across time.

The obvious advantage of a cross-sectional study is economy. One need not wait for 5-year-olds to become 6-year-olds, for single persons to get married, for nonsmokers to become smokers, and so forth. The compensating (and often overriding) disadvantage is that such a study does not lend itself well to developmental, much less causal, interpretations.

Example: A researcher interested in comparing the "young old" (age 65-75) with the "old old" (age greater than 75) is much more likely to carry out a cross-sectional rather than a longitudinal study of those two age groups. A longitudinal approach to such a study would carry the risk of subject mortality (in both the literal and the attritional sense of the word) in addition to being much more expensive in time and effort.

Cross-Tabulation

A cross-tabulation, often abbreviated to "cross-tab," is a two-way frequency distribution that expresses the bivariate relationship between two nominal or ordinal variables. Contingency table is a synonym for cross-tabulation and is a term preferred by some authors.

In a cross-tabulation, the frequency of occurrence of each combination of categories of the two variables is displayed in an i-by-j rectangular array, where i is the number of rows in the table (and therefore the number of categories for one of the variables) and j is the number of columns (the number of categories for the other variable). The "boxes" of the table that contain the actual frequencies are called cells. The row totals comprise the "marginal" frequency distribution for the first variable, and the column totals comprise the "marginal" frequency distribution for the second variable. These are almost always provided, along with the "grand total" (the sample size), so that the frequency distribution for each variable can be studied as well as the bivariate distribution.

Example: The relationship between sex and smoking behavior for a random sample of 200 people can be determined by displaying in a 2 (male/female)-by-2 (smoke/don't smoke) table the number of male smokers, female smokers, male nonsmokers, and female nonsmokers. The frequencies should also be converted into percentages to facilitate the proper interpretation of that relationship.

Cross-Validation

Cross-validation is a procedure that is sometimes carried out in connection with a regression analysis of the relationship between two variables.

What this usually entails is the splitting of the research sample (ideally randomly) into two parts (ideally equally), developing the appropriate regression equation for predicting Y from X for one half-sample, and comparing the predicted values of Y arising from that regression equation with the actual values of Y for the other half-sample for the same range of X values. The reason for this rather strange and complicated approach to studying the relationship between two variables is to avoid capitalization on the specific idiosyncrasies of a single sample that might produce an unreplicable pattern for a subsequent sample.

"Double" cross-validation is less common but equally feasible in the computer age. It involves the derivation of a regression equation for *each* half-sample and the comparison of the predicted values of Y arising from the equation for one half-sample with the actual values of Y for the other half-sample.

Example: The relationship between height and weight for a sample of 200 adult women might be studied by dividing the sample into two halves of 100 women each, regressing weight on height for one of the two half-samples, and comparing predicted weights with actual weights in the other half-sample to see how well the relationship determined in the first half-sample "holds up" under cross-validation.

C

Culture

There are many definitions of culture but no one standard or commonly accepted definition. Central to many definitions are notions of culture as (a) shared knowledge and customary patterns of behavior, (b) associated with groups of people who interact within a distinct social system or a subsystem of a larger society, (c) cumulative and symbolic in nature, and (d) transmitted from generation to generation. Description of culture or some aspect of culture is the purpose of ethnographic research.

See **Ethnography**.

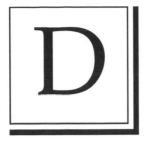

Data (Datum sing.)

Data *are* all of the pieces of information that are collected during a research study. The term *data* is plural, as its use in the preceding sentence suggests; *datum* is the singular form.

Database

A database is a collection of data that are organized to facilitate search and retrieval of information. Computerized databases are popular because of their storage capacities and the rapidity of search and retrieval. However, not all databases are computerized or need to be. The user determines the logic of the organizational scheme that will best serve data management needs.

Data Management

Data management is defined by Huberman and Miles (1994) as "the operations needed for a systematic, coherent process of data collection, storage, and retrieval" (p. 428). They stress the importance of designing an effective data management system prior to actual data collection. These authors are writing from the perspective of qualitative research, which typically generates large quantities of data. However, the concept is relevant for other researchers, since the need for a planned data management approach applies to any type of investigation.

Deductive Reasoning

Deductive reasoning is a way of thinking that is loosely described as moving from the general to the specific. A deductive theory building strategy consists of two premises and arrives at a conclusion that is dependent upon the premises:

(premise)	all A is B
(premise)	all C is A
(conclusion)	all C is B

The format is fixed, and therefore if the premises are faulty, the conclusion will be faulty as well.

A deductive research strategy begins with a general theory or set of abstract propositions that explains how variables of interest are related. To see if the explanations offered can be verified through empirical observation, a hypothesis is developed and variables are operationalized by indicating the observations that will generate appropriate empirical data for testing the hypothesis. (This is also called the hypothetico-deductive method.)

Deductive reasoning is closely associated with physical science, for example, physics and chemistry, and with mathematics. Some researchers believe that social/human sciences likewise should favor deductive approaches. But there are few instances of strictly deductive approaches to inquiry. Deduction is contrasted with induction. Theorists and researchers use both deduction and induction in their work.

See **Inductive Reasoning** and **Theory**.

Degrees of Freedom

Degrees of freedom is a technical term associated with sampling distributions such as t, F, and chi-square that are used in various tests of statistical significance. The number of degrees of freedom is one of the two reference points in tables for those distributions (level of significance is the other) that are found in the backs of just about all statistics books and some nursing research texts.

There are several ways of thinking about degrees of freedom, ranging from "something you need to carry out certain statistical tests" to "the number of unconstrained observations." Formulas for the number of degrees of freedom for a particular test vary considerably from one context to another, but they typically involve the sample size(s) and/or the number of variables.

See **Test of Significance**.

Delphi Technique

The Delphi technique is a method for obtaining expert opinion on a topic, for example, priorities in nursing research (Lindeman, 1975). It employs multiple "rounds" or "waves" of questionnaires, with each round utilizing information gathered during previous rounds, in an attempt to converge toward group consensus. It can best be thought of as intermediate between intensive interviewing and traditional survey research.

See Snyder-Halpern (1994) for an example of an application of the Delphi technique.

Dependent Samples

Dependent samples are samples that are "paired," "matched," or "correlated" in some manner.

The pairing can arise by virtue of the fact that the samples consist of the same people (or hospitals, thermometers, or whatever) measured on the dependent variable on more than one occasion. Alternatively, the samples may consist of different subjects who have been matched pairwise on the basis of one or more variables known or thought to be related to the dependent variable and are measured simultaneously on the dependent variable. The former situation occurs most often in nonexperimental longitudinal research and in "repeated-measures" experimental designs. The latter situation is common in "randomized-block" experimental designs, where each "block" is a pair of twins, a set of persons with identical or near-identical IQ scores, or the like.

Example: In studying the relative effectiveness of two types of aspirin regarding headache relief, a sample of *n* adults might be rank-ordered according to age, with one of the two oldest persons randomly assigned to Drug A and the other assigned to Drug B, one member of the next oldest pair randomly assigned to Drug A and the other to Drug B, and so on down through the youngest pair. The two samples would be dependent as they are matched on age.

D

Dependent Variable

The dependent variable in a research study is the variable that is of principal interest to the investigator, that is, the variable that really "counts." It is in contrast to the independent variable(s) that is (are) known or thought to be at least predictive if not actually causative of the dependent variable.

There is nothing special about *one* independent variable and *one* dependent variable. It is not unusual for a study, especially a nonexperimental study, to have as many as 10 or even 20 independent variables. An occasional study may also employ multiple dependent variables.

A given variable is not automatically relegated to one role or the other. The same measure that is used as the dependent variable in a particular study might very well serve as an independent variable in another study. Polit and Hungler (1991) illustrate that point in the following way: "a researcher may find that the religious background of a nurse (the independent variable) has an effect on his or her attitude toward death and dying (the dependent variable). Another study, however, may analyze the extent to which nurses' attitudes toward death and dying (the independent variables) affect their job performance (the dependent variable)" (p. 52).

Example: In a study of the effect of stress on depression, depression is the dependent variable that may be influenced by stress. Depression is the problem; stress may be symptomatic of, and/or lead to, depression.

Descriptive Research

Descriptive research is a type of quantitative research that is usually preliminary to more controlled experimental or correlational research. It provides a knowledge base when little is known about a phenomenon or when such things as clarification of a situation, classification of information, or description of subject characteristics will aid refinement of the research problem, formulation of hypotheses, or design of data collection and analysis procedures. Case studies and surveys are types of descriptive research. Descriptive research is not the same as qualitative research. Qualitative research, though descriptive or narrative in nature, is a cover term for a number of research traditions that are distinct in purpose, orientation, and design. They are discussed individually in this dictionary.

Descriptive Statistics

Descriptive statistics is the branch of statistics that is concerned with the summarization of data. The data may be for an entire population or for a sample.

Included under descriptive statistics are frequency distributions (the usual starting point for summarizing data), measures of central tendency (means, medians, modes), measures of variability (ranges, variances, standard deviations), measures of relationship (especially correlation coefficients), and various graphical techniques for displaying data.

For sample data, descriptive statistics are often used to highlight certain features of the data that will be the basis for making inferences from sample to population. However, when the data are for an entire population, the sole concern is with descriptive statistics, as there is no statistical inference to be made that goes beyond the data in hand.

Example: A sample survey of attitudes of student nurses toward homosexuality would have a very heavy descriptive statistical component, with frequency distributions for each item and each pair of items. Inferences regarding various population parameters might also be made, but the interpretation of the results of the survey will depend largely on the description of the sample data.

Design

In the broadest sense of the term, *design* refers to the portion of a research investigation that is concerned with sampling, operationalization of the constructs, decisions about and actual gathering of the data, and subjection of the data to analysis. In a narrower sense, the term applies to all of the methodological features *except* the measurement and the analysis, that is, those aspects of the research that come after problem specification and before data gathering and analysis. It should be noted, however, that for some kinds of research the design evolves as the research progresses.

Although design is often associated with the modifier "experimental," careful attention to design details is just as important in nonexperimental research as it is in experimental research. How are the subjects to be sampled? How many subjects are to be sampled? How is informed consent to be obtained? Are the subjects to be "debriefed"? These are just some of the design issues that must be faced in any kind of research that involves the explicit cooperation of human beings. The only important matter that is irrelevant for nonexperimental research is how the subjects are to be assigned to the treatment conditions, because there *are* no treatment conditions in research in which the principal independent variable is not manipulated.

Example: A researcher interested in the effect of anxiety on the academic achievement of student nurses must choose between an experimental design in which some student nurses are randomly assigned to an anxiety-producing condition and others are not, and a nonexperimental design in which anxiety is measured but not manipulated. One advantage of the experimental approach is that causal implications can be drawn. Advantages of the nonexperimental approach are that it is natural rather than artificial, is less threatening to the students, and is therefore more feasible.

Dialectic

Dialectic is from the Greek word that means "to converse," and the dialectic in Greek philosophy retains this sense of the term: a conversational form of argument; a method of explanation; a style of reasoning. Hegel used "the dialectic" to stand for the logical pattern that thought must follow, moving by contradiction and resolution of contradiction through reconciliation of opposing entities (thesis, antithesis, synthesis). Marxian theorists borrow from Hegel in asserting that change and development in nature and society occur in dialectical sequences of contradiction and synthesis, with reconciliation of contradictions producing new contradictions (the doctrine of dialectical materialism).

Critical theory-based research uses a methodology that is dialogical (pertaining to dialogue/conversation) and dialectical in nature.

See **Critical Theory**.

Dialogical Inquiry

Dialogical inquiry uses the metaphor of dialogue to express the way in which researchers engage in overlapping (simultaneously occurring) conversations (internal dialogue and dialogue with others) across systems of meaning and within the cultural systems of study participants. Embedded in the metaphor are a number of philosophical ideas about knowing and being, the nature of dialogue, and the structures that mediate communication.

The notion of dialogue emphasizes the reflective and cooperative nature of investigation. The researcher "dialogues" with the data. This reflective back-and-forth movement between the data and the interpretation produces insights about meaning. The imagery of dialogue also is used to describe data collection as an active two-way communication process between researchers and participants in relationships that are characterized by equality and mutuality. Padilla (1993), discussing the use of dialogical methods in group interviews, notes that the dialogue "redefines the purposes and outcomes of inquiry and recasts the roles of researchers and subjects in ways that lead to greater empowerment for the subjects" (p. 153). Dialogue creates the opportunity for participants to develop a critical understanding about problems in their lives, identify alternative options, and take action to improve their situation:

> The goal of the dialogical method is overtly political in the sense that its aim is to help subjects achieve a higher level of awareness about the sociopolitical structures and cultural practices that have shaped their lives. . . . [It], therefore, has its roots in a larger project of political freedom, cultural autonomy, and liberation from oppressive economic and social conditions. (Padilla, 1993, p. 154)

See **Critical Theory**.

Dichotomy

A dichotomy is a nominal variable that consists of just two categories.

Dichotomies are very common in nursing research, particularly as far as independent variables are concerned, because research questions regarding the relationships between sex (a male/female dichotomy) and depression, smoking behavior (a smoke/don't smoke dichotomy) and lung cancer, and the like, are of considerable interest. They are so popular that researchers often make the mistake of throwing away valuable data to get a dichotomy, for example, by collapsing age into two categories (say, under 65 and over 65) rather than keeping it as a continuum when studying its relationship with some dependent variable such as pulse rate.

Although dichotomies are nominal variables, they can be treated like interval variables in statistical calculations because the difference between the values assigned to the two categories constitutes a "unit" of measurement, however arbitrary, that is constant throughout the scale (it *is* the scale).

Example: Type of treatment (experimental/control) is the classic case of a dichotomy. In an experiment we are always interested in the

D

relationship between that variable and the dependent variable serving as a measure of the outcome of the experiment.

Discourse Analysis

Discourse analysis is an examination of language use—the assumptions that structure ways of talking and thinking about the topic of interest and the social functions that the discourse serves. It is a style of analysis linked with a branch of sociology (the sociology of knowledge) and with critical theory. As in critical theory, there is a focus on ideology and an intent to reveal how ideas and beliefs that underlie discourse are socially determined. In contrast, from a sociology of knowledge perspective, it need not be presumed that a particular factor such as social class or economy is preeminent over other possible causes for the shape that knowledge or belief takes in the discourse. And it is not presumed that the beliefs are necessarily true or false. The focus is on the relationship between knowledge and social structure. The assumption is that the social base produces certain kinds of knowledge that systematic and thoughtful analysis can reveal. There is particular interest in the ability of social discourse to close down conversation; that is, within a discourse there are things that cannot be said.

The work of Michel Foucault in this area has a distinct style and has been subject to various interpretations and criticisms. However, it has called attention to discourse analysis and the problems of discourse, as discussed in his *The Order of Things* (1966) and *The Archaeology of Knowledge* (1969). In separate works Foucault focused on knowledge, power, and the human body. In *Discipline and Punish* (1975) he explored aspects of power within prison systems. In *Madness and Civilization* (1961) he discussed ways of thinking and talking about madness. *The Birth of the Clinic* (1963) and *The History of Sexuality* (1976) were concerned with control of the body through use of certain forms of knowledge.

For additional information, see Hoy (1986), *Foucault: A Critical Reader*; Rabinow (1984), *The Foucault Reader*; and Sheridan (1980), *Michel Foucault: The Will to Truth*.

Discriminant Analysis

Discriminant analysis is a type of multivariate analysis in which two or more criterion groups defined according to some dependent variable are contrasted regarding two or more independent variables, to determine the extent to which those independent variables are capable of "discriminating" among the groups as far as prediction of group membership is concerned.

Discriminant analysis was used by Rizzuto, Bostrom, Suter, and Chenitz (1994) in their study of nurses' involvement in research activities.

See **Multivariate Analysis**.

Discriminant Validity

Discriminant validity is a type of construct validity. If there is *not* a strong relationship between a particular measure and one or more other measures that are alleged to operationalize different but easily confusable constructs, then the given measure is said to possess discriminant validity.

See **Validity**.

Double-Blind Study

A double-blind study is an experiment in which neither the experimenter nor the subject knows who is getting which treatment. (*Somebody*, usually the researcher who designs and analyzes the experiment, has to know or the data could never get sorted out.)

The purpose of the double-blind approach is to avoid the confounding of the actual treatment effect with any extraneous factors that may be associated with the mere knowledge of treatment identification, such as lack of motivation on the part of subjects who know that they have been given a placebo or the giving of additional encouragement to experimental subjects by the experimenter.

There are also "single-blind" experiments in which the subjects do not know which treatment they are receiving but the experimenters do.

Example: An experimental study of the effectiveness of any sort of pill, such as the every-other-day aspirin in The Physicians Health Study, often employs the double-blind technique. In that study the physicians were both subjects and experimenters, as they self-administered the pills that were mailed to them and they did not know whether they were getting the aspirin or the placebo.

Dummy Variable

A dummy variable is a special kind of dichotomy that uses the numbers 0 and 1 as codes to represent the two categories of the variable.

Dummy variables are most commonly used in conjunction with regression analysis, for natural dichotomies such as sex and type of treatment, and for artificial dichotomies arising from the coding of multicategoried nominal variables such as political affiliation and eye color. (Dummy coding is one of the three popular ways of coding; the other two are contrast coding and effect coding.)

Example: When investigating the relationship between attitude toward abortion (a continuous score of some kind) and religious affiliation (say a four-categoried nominal variable: Catholic, Protestant, Jew, Other), the religious affiliation variable might be transformed into three dummy variables X_1 (1 = Catholic, 0 = non-Catholic), X_2 (1 = Protestant, 0 = non-Protestant), and X_3 (1 = Jew, 0 = non-Jew), and a multiple regression analysis with those three independent variables and one dependent variable (the attitude score) carried out. A fourth dummy variable is both unnecessary and redundant, because the "Others" are uniquely identified by a coding of 0 on X_1, X_2, and X_3.

D

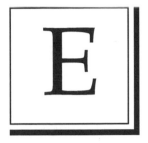

Effect Size

Effect size is a measure of an effect postulated in the alternative hypothesis, as contrasted with the "no effect" null hypothesis. It is usually defined as the difference between two population means divided by their common standard deviation. The term was coined by Jacob Cohen (1988) and is a crucial concept in the determination of sample size.

In the meta-analysis literature, effect size has a different meaning. There it is the *actual* effect obtained in a particular study, rather than a hypothesized effect.

The "effect" is not necessarily causal, no matter what the context.

Example: A researcher might hypothesize that the White/Black difference in intelligence (the effect size for skin color) is .5, that is, that the difference between the mean score for Whites and the mean score for Blacks on a typical intelligence test is half a standard deviation, which for a test such as the Stanford-Binet is eight IQ points.

Emic

This term relates to the perspectives that are shared and understood by members of a particular culture, the "insiders," in contrast to the perspectives of the culture that observers, the "outsiders," may have (etic perspectives). The contrast between emic and etic perspectives is important in ethnographic research.

See **Etic** and **Ethnography**.

Empirical Indicator/Referent

An empirical indicator or referent is an observable object, property, or event that is linked to a concept in a theory as a way of defining it.

See **Theory**.

Empirical Research

The term *empirical research* applies to any study in which some sort of evidence is obtained. The evidence is in turn called *data*. Empirical research is often confused with experimental research; the latter is a subset of the former.

See **Experiment** and **Research**.

Endogenous Variable

In path analysis an endogenous variable is any variable whose causal determination is of interest to the researcher and the nature of that causation is hypothesized in the path model.

See **Path Analysis**.

Epidemiological Research

Epidemiological research is a strategy for trying to determine the causes, both necessary and sufficient, for the distribution and rates of occurrence of disease phenomena in human populations. It is a relatively new approach to causal inference in nursing research but warrants more attention than it has so far received in doctoral programs and from practicing researchers.

Although it is not a type of research in the same sense that experimental research and survey research are, epidemiological research is a very special way of advancing knowledge. Epidemiology as a substantive discipline is the study of diseases in human populations. Epidemiologists use the term *disease* in its broadest sense to include social problems such as suicide, drug abuse, and abortion. Causal inferences in epidemiological research are almost never based on controlled experiments, as the kinds of independent variables of principal concern in such research usually are not manipulable. The "case-control" type of retrospective research is the approach most commonly employed. (See Kleinbaum, Kupper, & Morgenstern, 1982, and Ryan, 1983, for further discussion of these matters.)

Example: A research question that lends itself very nicely to this sort of approach is given by Ryan (1983): "Does use of side rails prevent or increase the likelihood of falls in the elderly?" Although that sounds like a "natural" for a controlled experiment, it may be unethical or impractical to randomly assign half of a group of elderly persons to beds that have side rails and randomly assign the other half to beds that are not so equipped. In addition to this general question regarding side rails, there are other interesting questions that also need to be addressed, such as (again Ryan, 1983):

1. What characteristics are common to those who fall?
2. What characteristics are associated with *only* those who fall?
3. How often do people fall, with or without side rails?
4. How serious are the injuries that result from falls?

Epistemology

Epistemology is a concept in philosophy that relates to theories of knowledge or how people come to have knowledge of the world. In discussions about theory building and research, the term is used to refer to particular perspectives in scientific methods that lead to acquisition of knowledge in a discipline. For example, human science perspectives and methods have a different epistemology from those that are based on the concepts, worldview, and techniques of natural science.

EQS

EQS is a computer package that is used in structural equation modeling, and is generally favored over LISREL by "West Coast" researchers.

An application of the use of EQS to test a theoretical model is given by Lusk, Ronis, Kerr, and Atwood (1994).

See **LISREL** and **Structural Equation Modeling**.

Error

The term *error* is used in several contexts in nursing research but usually does not refer to making a mistake.

One of the most common contexts is in the analysis of variance, where error refers to within-treatment variance attributable to individual differences among subjects who receive the same experimental treatment, but do not get the same score on the dependent variable. Another context is in sampling, where a particular statistic for a

51

sample is not exactly equal to the corresponding population parameter because of chance factors associated with the drawing of the sample. A third context is classical measurement theory, where a measurement error is defined as the difference between an "obtained" score and a "true" score.

The one context in which the term "error" actually means mistake is in statistical hypothesis-testing. A "Type I error" is the rejection of a true null hypothesis; a "Type II error" is the failure to reject a false null hypothesis.

Essences

In phenomenology, essences constitute meaning of an experience as lived, that is, what it is like for different individuals or for one individual: "Eidetic [descriptive] phenomenology as a research method rests on the thesis that there are essential structures to any human experience. . . . When these structures are apprehended in consciousness, they take on a meaning that is the meaning (or truth) of that experience for the participants" (Cohen & Omery, 1994, pp. 147-148).

See **Phenomenology**.

Ethnography

Ethnography is a qualitative research approach developed by anthropologists. It is both a process and a product, the purpose of which is to describe a culture or particular aspects of a culture. As a process it involves an attitude inclined toward learning from rather than studying people. The aim is to capture "the native's point of view" (Malinowski, 1922, p. 25). To grasp the way members of a cultural group envision their world (their worldview) and see themselves in relation to others constitutes what is called an emic approach—that is, it is concerned with ways that "insiders" experience and interpret life in contrast to an "outsider," or etic, view of what the culture is like. Ethnographers analyze both emic and etic perspectives together in order to capture differences between what people say and what they do.

Ethnographic work is rooted in some concept of culture. Culture is defined in various ways, for example, as customary practices or patterns of behavior; in relation to social structure, lifeways, values, rituals and beliefs, products, and artifacts; or as knowledge acquired through generations that guides people's actions and is used by them to interpret their experiences. An implicit principle in ethnographic research is that the best instrument to use in understanding cultural systems and themes is human, as in the expression "the researcher is the instrument." That is, the researcher can only capture an "insider" point of view through some degree of immersion in the culture. The quality of the research depends on the nature and extent of personal involvement and the success with which the researcher can (a) combine intellectual skills of objective reasoning with subjective reflection and human qualities of empathy, caring, and sensitivity; and (b) explicitly bring all of these dimensions to bear on the research both while it is in process and when it is presented in finished form.

Knowledge of a culture is gained through fieldwork, a method that requires the researcher's presence in the cultural environment—living and participating in everyday life, systematically recording and validating observations, and interviewing. Participant observation is the central technique used in fieldwork. It involves engaging in everyday activities for the explicit purpose of systematically observing their nature, the people who participate, and the context in which the activities take place.

A variety of data-gathering techniques is used in conjunction with participant observation. Intensive (in-depth) interviewing employs a conversational style to draw individuals out and allow them to talk at great length on a topic. Conversation combines open-ended and structured interview formats to varying degrees. In cases where strong emotions, sensitive issues, and strongly held values are involved, the interview style allows the researcher to gently and deeply probe for what might be difficult to obtain from ordinary conversation or more formal interview styles.

Key-informant interviewing involves selective use of members of the culture who are especially knowledgeable, insightful, and articulate or who have specialized knowledge not shared by the rest of the community. Because such personal views are distorted by individual history, key-informant interviewing is used as a supplement to participant observation and other techniques.

Life history is another technique that involves the recounting of the stories of key informants' lives in great detail. Life histories can help to place in perspective the interplay between individuals and culture across the life span.

Ethnoscience (semantic ethnography) is yet another approach to understanding culture, by analyzing native language categories. It is based on the assumption that people's worldviews are reflected in speech. However, a clear association between categories of cognition (how people think) and categories of language (how people classify objects and events) has not been demonstrated.

Standard techniques of systematic observation, questionnaires, and administration of projective psychological tests may be used. Collection of various items of material culture or commonly used substances, such as medicinal plants, provides other views of lifeways of a people. And technological approaches—photography, film, audio-taping—help to capture visual and auditory images.

Unlike other research methods where data are first collected and then analyzed, ethnographic fieldnotes are continuously analyzed for answers to questions that naturally occur as the researcher attempts to understand what is happening. But most important is the search for questions not yet asked or thought about in relation to the social situation under study. The process of question discovery—learning the questions most relevant to the setting—is what moves the investigation forward through numerous cycles of experiencing, observing, asking questions, listening and recording, and analyzing until the research is complete. Participant observers who approach field research as a disciplined and repeated cycling of recording and analyzing data know when they have sufficient information on any topic; have distinguished background description from study focus; and have combed through the data for unanswered questions. Consequently, they are not so likely to be overwhelmed by a mass of unorganized narrative. They have evolved a system of coding, arranging, and reflecting on what is present in the fieldnotes before the written account begins to take shape. And they have achieved a balance between personal involvement and participation in the culture to obtain an insider point of view *and* a degree of intellectual detachment and distancing that is required for analysis and written reports. They continuously make mental shifts back and forth between the demands of the participant and the observer roles to view what they are learning from as many perspectives as possible.

Fieldnotes themselves do not constitute a description of culture. They become the source within which knowledge of culture is embedded—hence the emphasis on adequacy of the description, attention to accuracy and detail, and a disciplined and systematic approach. There are aspects of culture that are readily observable and can be explicitly communicated by study participants, for example, customs, routine practices, linguistic expressions, and characteristic social expectations. However, the aim of continuous analysis of the data throughout the time in the field is to draw out themes and insights that are both explanatory and predictive of what may be the tacit taken-for-granted understandings that guide people's actions and shape their beliefs, that is, underlying values and assumptions. This involves making inferences about what people say, what they do, the consistency between what they say and what they do, and what it all means within the context in which everyday activities and interactions are taking place.

Ethnography as a product of ethnographic fieldwork and participant observation is cultural description. But the writing of ethnography is an interpretive task. It involves both description of cultural patterns that includes the empirical evidence (descriptive details) from which the patterns were drawn *and* translation of what the patterns mean to people in that particular social situation in such a way that individuals with a different cultural perspective can readily understand. Ethnographic work that describes cultural patterns without interpretation of what the patterns mean is incomplete.

A process of generalization is central to the task of writing ethnography. The necessity to make general statements about what the culture is like and to support those statements with examples representing the empirical evidence on which they are based is only partially dictated by the need to reduce and summarize large masses of data into a more manageable form. The greater necessity for generalization involves a search for underlying patterns, themes, rules, or assumptions that produces abstractions representative of meaning structures, that is, the ethnographer's interpretive account or literary translation of what people express through and derive from culture and its effect on their lives.

Accuracy—providing a true and balanced account of a culture—is the major goal of ethnographic writing. Readers need to be told how the fieldwork was conducted and what important variables might be affecting the culture (e.g., historical events, political and economic conditions, the effect of the researcher's presence); aspects of the culture to which the researcher did or did not have access; conditions under which data were obtained; and techniques used. This is only a sample of what should be communicated so that a reader can judge the quality of the research and the likelihood of producing similar findings were the research to be repeated. The process of generalization used in analyzing data and producing the written accounts also needs to be explained. Reports should indicate what the evidence supporting generalized statements (summaries and abstractions) consists of, for example, observations, interviews, or shared experi-

E

ences. The analytical process followed (e.g., how data were sorted into categories, compared, and contrasted) and the link between conclusions and empirical evidence should be clear to the reader. Ethnographic reports vary a great deal in how much of this sort of information is provided. Sometimes this is attributable to the limited space in scientific journals and the emphasis on conciseness and efficiency that precludes the fullness of description required to answer all of the questions readers might have. In instances where there is not enough information to judge the accuracy of the account, the reader must apply a more intuitive criterion, namely that of credibility—considering if, given what is already known of a culture, the account makes sense and is believable.

Although journal articles are a major means of scholarly communication, they allow for only limited or specialized treatment of data from ethnographic projects. The ethnographic description of a culture cannot be confined to space available in this type of format. Anthropologists, therefore, often use the longer monograph (book) as a standard medium for reporting ethnographic research. However, there is no standard style of ethnographic writing. Representation of a culture may range from abstract generalizations to highly personal accounts. Ethnographies (monographs) and shorter ethnographic reports may emphasize theoretical issues or read like a novel, complete with a cast of characters and a variety of plots or scenarios that illustrate what life in the culture is like. Much depends on the purpose of the written piece—the message the writer wishes to convey, the audience for whom it is intended, and the effect the writer wishes to produce. Ethnographic research is a craft. The personal skills and preferences as well as the professional orientations and intellectual interests of researchers affect the organization, language, and communication style used in the written report. All of the styles should be studied and appreciated as efforts to sharpen and extend researchers' human capacities to understand the worldviews of other people.

For additional information on ethnography, see Aamodt (1991); Atkinson (1992); Boyle (1994); Hughes (1992); Kleinman (1992); Muecke (1994); Stein (1991); and Van Maanen (1988).

For research examples in nursing, see Connelly, Keele, Kleinbeck, Schneider, and Cobb (1993); Dombeck (1991); Lipson (1991a); Magilvy, Congdon, and Martinez (1994); Miller (1991); Powers (1988a, 1988b, 1991, 1992); Rempusheski (1988); and Tripp-Reimer, Sorofman, Lauer, Martin, and Afifi (1988).

Ethnomethodology

Ethnomethodology (literally, "people's methods") is a branch of sociology created by Harold Garfinkel in the 1940s. Its aim is to study how people "do" everyday things (initiate telephone conversations, walk, invite laughter, and deal with unexpected disruptions in the daily flow of their lives). The last example represents a type of study, the breaching experiment, for which ethnomethodology gained some notoriety. For example, Garfinkel asked his students to behave as if they were boarders while they were at home, and to note family members' reactions. In another demonstration, students were instructed to select a non-family member, and, in the course of conversation, to bring their faces close to the subject until their noses almost touched. Of interest were the ways in which people tried to cope with such breaches in usual expected behavior. Another type of investigation involved conversational analysis (e.g., telephone talk, courtroom conversation) to observe how people used language to create some sort of order in social settings. The assumption is that people work continuously to manage and make sense of their everyday lives, but the way in which the social world is thus constructed is completely taken for granted.

Ethnomethodology originated as a critique of mainstream sociology. Traditional sociologists were accused of imposing their views of social reality on the social world rather than being attentive to subjects' views. Further, sociologists' reliance on coding techniques, statistical analysis of data, and abstract descriptions of findings were thought to distort the social world in major ways. Traditional sociology views people as being shaped and constrained by external forces. Ethnomethodology views people as creators and shapers of social reality through their thoughts and actions; that is, reality is reflexive activity. Reality is not "out there." It is created through human interaction; and it is coherent and organized, permeable (people live within a variety of social worlds and move easily between them on a day-to-day basis), and fragile (taken-for-granted social realities are prone to disruption and to the unexpected—or can be disrupted as demonstrated by the breaching experiments). (See Mehan & Wood, 1975, p. 6.)

Ethnomethodologists gather empirical data through observation, conversation, and video or audio recording, not to describe everyday life but to theorize about the nature of structuring activities in which people engage and the taken-for-granted use of rules in social situations. The late 1960s and early 1970s was a productive period for

E

ethnomethodologists in terms of published research: Sudnow (1967), *Passing On: The Social Organization of Dying*; Garfinkel (1967), *Studies in Ethnomethodology*; Cicourel (1968), *The Social Organization of Juvenile Justice*; McHugh (1968), *Defining the Situation*; and MacAndrew and Edgerton (1969), *Drunken Comportment*. However, debate within sociology generated sufficient criticism of this movement to hinder its spread, and practitioners became dispersed and absorbed into other areas of study within the discipline. Some nurse sociologists have a background in ethnomethodology, but it has not been influential as a research trend within nursing. In the passage of time there have been splits among ethnomethodologists over favored research styles (e.g., conversational analysis vs. rule-use analysis); and it is difficult for "outsiders" to determine when reading the general sociological literature if a person's work actually reflects an ethnomethodological position (Mullins, 1973). Consequently, its transition to specialty status in the 1980s was impeded, and it would seem to be a fading trend with a scattering of adherents whose insights will be passed on to students whose current options in terms of research orientations are more numerous and varied.

Ethnoscience

Ethnoscience (semantic ethnography) is a method of analyzing culture to ascertain the system of knowledge and beliefs as it is reflected in native-language categories. It focuses on emic ("insider") data. Results are often in the form of taxonomies or semantic network diagrams.

See **Emic**, **Ethnography**, and **Etic**.

Etic

This term relates to the perspectives of a culture held by observers who are "outsiders" or nonparticipants themselves. The contrast between "insider" and "outsider" views (emic vs. etic) is of concern in ethnographic research.

See **Emic** and **Ethnography**.

Evaluation Research

Evaluation research is a term that is applied to a wide spectrum of investigative activities that employ research methods and a problem-solving process to meet program or practice needs. In institutional settings another term used for this type of research is quality assurance.

In nursing, as in other practice disciplines, the term *evaluation* is associated with processes for assessing and judging the quality of care or services rendered. In the health sciences this is a very important—and legally mandated—activity that may focus on structure, for example, the effectiveness of programs, policies, and procedures; on process, e.g., the quality of practitioner performance; or on outcome, e.g., the effect(s) of a particular type of care or service on recipients. The usual approach involves identifying criteria or behavioral objectives that represent the goals, valued practice models, or desired outcomes; setting a "standard" that represents the level (often expressed as a percentage) at which each criterion must be met in order to judge the program, policy, procedure, practice, and so forth as "effective" or of "acceptable quality"; employing data collection and analysis methods designed to answer the question about the extent of compliance with the standard set for each criterion (this could involve experimental or nonexperimental methodologies); implementing corrective changes if indicated; and setting the cycle in motion again by evaluating the results. (A standard must not be confused with a norm. A norm is "what is"; a standard is "what should be.")

Evaluation can be formative or summative. Formative evaluation allows for continuous feedback and adjustment of interventions or programs as they progress. The emphasis is on monitoring them as they develop. Summative evaluation focuses on how a program or practice influences the outcomes that the study seeks to measure, that is, how effective it is in meeting stated objectives or standards.

See **Applied Research.**

Ex Post Facto Research

Although the term *ex post facto research* is used in a number of different ways in nursing research (some authors equate it with any form of nonexperimental research), it is best thought of as a retrospective type of causal-comparative correlational research.

In ex post facto research one starts with the dependent variable and makes a search into the past for one or more independent variables that may at least partially "explain" that dependent variable.

Example: The prototypical example of ex post facto research is the investigation of the association between cigarette smoking and lung cancer. Such an investigation most often begins by identifying a group of people who have lung cancer and a comparable group who do not have lung cancer, and proceeds to attempt to determine if the cigarette-smoking history for the two groups differs. If the cancer group

E

has a long history of heavy smoking and the "control" group (that designation is often used even though the study is *not* an experiment) does not, a case can be made that cigarette smoking is one of the possible causes of lung cancer. It is essential to realize, however, that such evidence does not prove that cigarette smoking *is* an actual cause, much less the only cause.

Exogenous Variable

In path analysis an exogenous variable is any variable whose causative determination is external to the path model and is of no interest to the researcher.

See **Path Analysis**.

Experiment

An experiment is a study that involves manipulation of the principal independent variable, that is, the actual administration of treatments or interventions that comprise the categories of the independent variable. An investigation is made of the effect of the independent variable on the dependent variable.

A true experiment is characterized by a high degree of control over the unwanted influence of extraneous variables and other factors that could bias the results of the study. The researcher typically investigates the difference on the dependent variable between one group of subjects who get the experimental treatment and another group of subjects who do not. (It sometimes happens that the experimental group and the control group consist of the *same* people, i.e., every person gets *both* the experimental treatment *and* the control treatment, in randomized order. Such designs are called repeated-measures designs.)

In some experiments the dependent variable is measured both before and after the intervention. The measurement taken before the intervention is called a pretest and the measurement taken after the intervention is called a posttest. In other experiments the measurement is taken only after the intervention. The former designs are called, naturally enough, "pretest-posttest designs," whereas the latter designs are called "posttest-only designs."

In an experiment involving two (or more) independent variables, one may be interested not only in the effect of each of them on the dependent variable but also in the combined effect (interaction) of the independent variables. Experimental designs in which both kinds of effects are tested are called factorial designs.

Example: A study in which one group of nursing students is taught how to administer an injection by Teaching Method A (a film, say) and another group of students is taught by Method B ("hands-on" demonstration using a dummy, say), is an experiment because the principal independent variable (type of teaching method) is actually manipulated by the researcher.

Experimental Group

The experimental group is the group that receives the "treatment" of particular interest to the researcher.

See **Experiment**.

Exploratory Data Analysis

Exploratory data analysis is a type of statistical analysis that utilizes a special collection of largely graphical descriptive statistics for summarizing research findings.

Included under exploratory data analysis are techniques such as stem-and-leaf diagrams and q-q plots that lend themselves very nicely to modern-day computer technology. (For further details see Tukey, 1977; Jacobsen, 1981; and three articles by Ferketich and Verran—Ferketich & Verran, 1986; Verran & Ferketich, 1987a, 1987b.)

Example: One of Tukey's popular statistics is the "95% trimmed mean," which is the mean for a particular variable calculated after the highest 2½% and the lowest 2½% of the observations have been deleted (trimmed). The rationale for this is to determine an average that is not affected by extreme data ("outliers") that might otherwise have an undue influence. Such a statistic is routinely reported in statistical "packages" that include exploratory data analyses.

External Validity

External validity is a synonym for generalizability, which is one of the important goals of most scientific research.

The term was coined by Campbell and Stanley (1966) in their classic work on experimental designs. A study is said to have a high degree of external validity if the results of the study can be generalized to people, measuring instruments, settings, and so forth other than the ones actually employed in the study itself. Campbell and Stanley (1966) discuss a number of "threats" to the external validity of a research design that might restrict its generalizability, for example, "reactive arrangements" such as the Hawthorne Effect whereby people who know they are participating in a research study may behave differently from the way they would behave in "real life."

"External validity" is actually an unfortunate choice of term for this characteristic of a research investigation, because the root word *validity* is a *measurement* term that may have nothing at all to do with generalizability.

Example: A study of the effect of previous information about patients on the attitudes of student nurses toward those patients would have greater external validity if two sets of descriptions (one favorable, one unfavorable) were randomly distributed to the students without telling them that they were part of a study, than if they were told. Such a study might raise some ethical questions, however, because the students would be manipulated without either their knowledge or their consent.

Extraneous Variable

An extraneous variable is a potentially confounding variable that is not of any particular interest to the researcher, but should be controlled if the results of the study are to be interpreted properly.

See **Control**.

E

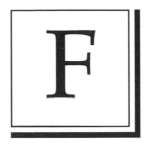

F Test

The *F* test is a test of statistical significance that is usually associated with the analysis of variance.

Gulick (1994) carried out several *F* tests in conjunction with her factorial analysis of variance.

See **Test of Significance.**

Face Validity

Face validity is a type of content validity in which the "expert" judgment of the validity of an instrument is provided by the people who are to be measured with the instrument.

See **Validity.**

Factor Analysis

Factor analysis is a statistical procedure for determining the underlying dimensionality of a set of variables.

The variables can be as specific as a collection of test items or as general as a group of physiological measurements. In the former case the focus is typically on the subscale structure (whether or not there *are* subscales, and if so, *how many* subscales are necessary to describe the construct being measured). In the latter case it is often a matter of trying to cut down on the number of variables by arriving at the most "parsimonious" factor solution.

Most factor analyses are "exploratory" in that no theoretical expectations are formulated beforehand as to the number or nature of underlying factors. The most common such procedure is the so-called Little Jiffy technique that involves principal components factor extraction with orthogonal rotation to simple structure of all factors for which the eigenvalues are greater than one. (See Harris, 1985, or almost any other textbook on multivariate analysis for technical details.) Some factor analyses are "confirmatory" in that certain hypotheses regarding the number of factors and the factor structure are actually tested in the process of carrying out the analysis. The distinction between exploratory and confirmatory factor analysis is summarized in Munro and Page's (1993) text.

Example: An exploratory factor analysis of a 100-item health behavior inventory might yield two subscales that could be identified as "Beliefs" and as "Practices," with some items contributing primarily to the Belief dimension and with other items contributing primarily to the Practices dimension.

Factorial Design

A factorial design is a design that involves two or more independent variables whose main effects and interaction effects are of equal interest in the research. The term is usually associated with experimental research in which the independent variables are actually manipulated by the investigator.

See **Interaction Effect** and **Main Effect**.

Feasibility Study

A feasibility study is a small-scale study that is undertaken to determine if the design, instrumentation, and analysis for the proposed "main study" are practicable. The results of such a study are of no concern. The focus is on the extent to which the logistical features of the proposed study are capable of being carried out successfully.

A feasibility study is similar to a pilot study, although the latter type of study is often used to gather some preliminary evidence regarding the validity and the reliability of the measuring instruments.

Example: A main study in which very expensive and/or invasive instrumentation is to be employed should be preceded by a feasibility study whose principal objective is to see if research subjects will be willing to be "attached" to various devices, how much time it will take to gather the data, and the like.

Feminist Methodology

Feminist methodology involves an epistemological stance, or way of looking at the world, that gives direction to the diversity of evolving research practices in this field. The goal is to entertain a critical dialogue that focuses on women's experiences in historical, cultural, and socioeconomic perspective.

Lather (1991) asserts that "to do feminist research is to put the social construction of gender at the center of one's inquiry" (p. 71). The use of gender as an organizing principle informs research practice in a variety of ways. First, priority is given to the pervasive influence of gender in everyday life, with women as the focus of analysis. The emphasis on female experience takes into account the central role that men have played in understanding human behavior. The major assumption of feminist criticism is that in the enterprise of knowledge development through theory and research, either women have been ignored or their experiences have been distorted and misunderstood as a result of interpreting them from a masculine point of view. Stressing female alienation in a male-dominated world enables feminist scholars to illuminate women's realities and to identify tensions and contradictions arising from gender asymmetry that suggest a need for alternative approaches and new understandings.

Second, consciousness raising, as a central theme in feminist methodology, maintains attention on gender issues. There are several ways in which this occurs. Consciousness raising may be an outcome of the effect of the research on feminist researchers themselves. That is, the increased awareness and insight acquired through their work in the research process may produce a heightened sensitivity to women's perspectives and concerns. Research participants also may experience consciousness raising as a result of their involvement in the research. "Some authors view the research act as an explicit attempt to reduce the distance between the woman researcher and female subjects" (Fonow & Cook, 1991, p. 3). Additionally, consciousness-raising techniques, such as role playing and group discussion, often are used in data gathering to explore women's collective consciousness and encourage validation of shared experience. The intent of consciousness raising is empowerment of women to bring about change in their own lives as well as encouragement of social and political action on behalf of women. "This emphasis on action is something feminists share

F

with other traditions of social thought such as Black Studies, Marxism, and Gay and Lesbian Studies" (Fonow & Cook, 1991, p. 5).

Finally, feminist epistemology draws attention to the affective dimension of research. Attending to emotions that emerge within the context of the research is part of the critical reflexivity (emphasis on reflection and critical analysis) that guides approaches to knowledge. This means that themes related to caring and emotional attachment among participants and between the researcher and the researched are discussed and analyzed. There also is a similar tendency to address the meaning of negative emotions evoked by, or occurring in the course of, the research process.

Feminist scholars' engagement around ethical issues in research includes concerns about the personal welfare of participants and perspectives about researchers' and participants' mutual creation of data. For example, they have questioned the ethics of withholding information and assistance from participants and have intervened and used collaborative strategies in conducting research. Researchers differ in terms of the extent and nature of participant involvement in research. Some, in an effort to avoid exploitation of women as research objects and to empower them to pursue particular issues, have identified study participants as co-researchers. In other instances, participants may be asked to read and comment on portions of the data analysis. Olesen (1994) observes that negotiating new participatory forms in research "in consultation with participants, rather than as an afterthought, challenges feminist researchers at many levels," including:

> Assumptions about women's knowledge; representations of women; modes of data gathering, analysis, interpretation, and writing the account; relationships between researcher and participants and, critically, diversity among women's views about women, particularly where views are not similar to feminist outlooks (Hess, 1990); and the risk of appropriating participant-generated data to or along the lines of the researcher's interests (Opie, 1992). (pp. 166-167)

Feminist researchers use the techniques and strategies of qualitative and quantitative methods to design studies oriented to the epistemological concerns discussed above. However, Hall and Stevens (1991) note that although "conventional quantitative methods may be employed . . . it is not likely that conventional quantitative methods alone will be adequate for studies of women's lived experiences"

(p. 26). Their discussion of rigor in feminist research includes a critique of conventional empiricist criteria of reliability and validity and suggests more appropriate concepts to use in evaluating the scientific adequacy of feminist research. These concepts include (a) reflexivity—knowledge is jointly constructed by researchers and research participants; (b) credibility—descriptions of women's experiences are understandable and believable; (c) rapport—researchers are involved with participants in relationships of trust and openness; (d) coherence—research conclusions are logically consistent with data; (e) complexity—research emphasizes the context and reflects the complexity of reality; (f) consensus—the researcher deals with variety and seeks consensus in accounts of women's experiences by searching for recurring themes, negative cases, divergent experiences, and alternative explanations; (g) relevance—questions address women's concerns, and answers to the questions serve women's interests; (h) honesty and mutuality—ethical issues of honesty are stressed, there are efforts to reduce power inequalities in researcher-participant relationships, and feedback and assistance that might be useful to participants are offered; (i) naming—research reports pay attention to language, feature women's voices, and avoid androcentric concepts; and (j) relationality—collaboration with other scholars as well as with members of groups being studied is encouraged.

Some examples of feminist methodology in nursing literature include (a) Thompson's (1991) participatory feminist approach to exploring psychosocial adjustment and gender issues in a support group for Khmer refugee women; (b) White's (1991) critical analysis of traditional biomedical and psychiatric approaches to eating disorders in women; (c) MacPherson's (1992) critical analysis of the biomedical model definition of cardiovascular disease in women and the debates about noncontraceptive use of hormones; (d) P. E. Stevens's (1993, 1994) narrative analysis about protective strategies used by marginalized women and their access to health care, involving focus groups and individual interviews in a multicultural metropolitan lesbian community; (e) Montgomery's (1994) grounded theory feminist analysis of the strengths and personal resources of women who survive homelessness; (f) Hall's (1994a, 1994b) ethnographic interview study of how lesbians, one specific at-risk population, recognize and respond to alcohol problems; (g) Caroline and Bernhard's (1994) critical literature review and conceptualization of health-related risks for women with serious mental illness; and (h) Howell's (1994) grounded theory study of women with chronic nonmalignant pain.

Although individual studies differ in focus and the extent to which various concerns of feminist epistemology are addressed, the common assumption is that knowledge produced through feminist research can be used by women to challenge misunderstandings and to change oppressive and exploitative social conditions. Campbell and Bunting (1991), in contrasting similarities of and differences between the emancipatory paradigms of feminist theory and critical theory, discuss how history and epistemology influence the methodology that is distinctive of feminist research:

> Feminist theory has the primary goal of presenting a women-centered patterning of human experience. . . . Even though contemporary critical theorists are now broadening their approach to include gender issues, gender is not central in critical theory. . . . [And] both [feminist and critical theorists] agree that social structures can and have resulted in class oppression, but feminists choose division and domination according to gender as the fundamental oppression. (Campbell & Bunting, 1991, pp. 9-10)

F

This idea that feminist theory and research are *for* rather than about women is central to understanding feminist methodology as a whole. However, it is equally important to understand that there is no method unique to feminist research (Harding, 1987). Feminist studies likely will continue as a highly differentiated field of specialization, influenced and enhanced by diverse schools of thought and multiple innovative as well as traditional research strategies.

See also the *Advances in Nursing Science* (1991, volume 13, number 3) issue on "Feminism and Nursing" as well as Bunting and Campbell (1990) for a historical perspective on feminism and nursing; DeMarco, Campbell, and Wuest (1993) for history and implications of using feminist critique as a mode of inquiry; Pohl and Boyd (1993) for a discussion of ageism within feminism; and Nielsen (1990) for readings in the social sciences.

Fieldnotes

Fieldnotes are written detailed descriptions of researchers' observations, experiences, and conversations in the "field," that is, research setting. Most fieldworkers write these notes from memory, but sometimes audiotaping is used. Space should be left on each page of ongoing description for later coding and analytic notes. Also, the researcher's subjective comments need to be easily distinguishable from descriptive data. Many ethnographers keep a separate personal journal in which they record their thoughts, feelings, questions, hunches, and ideas.

Sanjek (1990) discusses different approaches to producing and working with fieldnotes in his edited volume *Fieldnotes: The Makings of Anthropology.*

See **Fieldwork** and **Ethnography**.

Fieldwork

Fieldwork is an anthropological research approach that traditionally involves prolonged residence with members of the culture that is being studied. Field methods are also used by researchers across disciplines working within other research traditions (e.g., grounded theory). Modified field approaches do not always involve residence with study participants. But they do require the researcher to conduct the research in the natural settings that are familiar to informants and to incorporate knowledge of the setting into the research plan.

Fieldwork associated with ethnographic research does not necessarily require relocation to a foreign setting. It can take place in small villages or large cities, restaurants or bus stations, hospitals or schools. The researcher can travel a distance or turn to something close at hand. The consistent requirements are that (a) the research involves a social situation that can be described in terms of a physical setting, people who are associated with and interact in the setting, and patterns of activity from which a cultural accounting can be drawn; and (b) the researcher is prepared to become personally involved within the setting in a rather time-intensive effort. On one hand, it is frequently recommended that novice researchers, in particular, immerse themselves in a situation that is unfamiliar to them. The advantage is thought to be that there is little that the researcher can take for granted and therefore the tendency to impose already formed assumptions on the data will be reduced. On the other hand, in settings that are familiar to researchers, there must be a self-conscious heightening awareness of what is taking place to account for information that insiders might normally screen out, for example, certain sounds, sights, actions, and expressions taken as usual, routine, and "what everybody already knows."

For discussion of the fieldworker role, see Boyle (1991), "Field Research: A Collaborative Model for Practice and Research"; Field (1991), "Doing Fieldwork in Your Own Culture"; Lipson (1991b), "The

F

Use of Self in Ethnographic Research"; and Rew, Bechtel, and Sapp (1993), "Self-as-Instrument in Qualitative Research."

For examples of fieldwork experience, see Kauffman (1994) and Kidd (1992).

See **Ethnography**.

Focus Groups

Focus groups generate data on a designated topic through discussion and interaction. Sessions are moderated by a group leader and are conducted as informal semistructured interviews. Often group interviews are used in conjunction with other interviewing and observation techniques. However, they can be used as primary data collection methods. Participants are systematically selected on the basis of their ability to provide the most meaningful information on the topic.

See Morgan and Zhao (1993) for an example of the use of focus groups to investigate the doctor-caregiver relationship and Saint-Germain, Bassford, and Montano (1993) for comparison of the findings from two studies (survey vs. focus group interviews) on barriers to health care use in general and to breast cancer screening in particular with older Hispanic women.

Useful resources on planning and conducting focus groups and on analyzing focus group data include Carey (1994); Carey and Smith (1994); Kingry, Tiedje, and Friedman (1990); Krueger (1994); and Morgan (1993).

Frequency Distribution

A frequency distribution is a count of each of the different values for a variable. Most frequency distributions are "univariate," that is, for one variable at a time. But bivariate (and even multivariate) frequency distributions are of considerable interest as they provide counts for cross-tabulations of values that give some indication of the relationships between variables.

Perhaps the most important frequency distribution in the study of statistics is the theoretical "normal," or bell-shaped, distribution for which most of the values are in the center of the distribution and very few are located at the extremes. Other important frequency distributions are the t, F, and chi-square sampling distributions that are used in inferential statistics.

Frequency distributions are often characterized according to their degrees of "skewness" and "kurtosis." A distribution that has several observations (a "hump") at the low end of the scale and very few (a "tail") at the high end of the scale is called *positively* skewed, or skewed to the right, whereas a distribution that is heavy at the high end and light at the low end is called *negatively* skewed, or skewed to the left. A distribution that has an unusually large concentration of scores near the middle of the distribution is referred to as *leptokurtic;* if the distribution is "flat" with approximately equal frequencies throughout the scale, it is called *platykurtic;* and the intermediate case is *mesokurtic.*

Example: A frequency distribution of the birth years of residents in a nursing home who are the subjects of a gerontological study would show not only how the group breaks down between the "young old" and the "old old" but how many people there are in the study within each of those divisions.

Fundamental Research
  See **Basic Research** and **Research**.

F

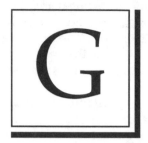

G

Generalizations

Generalizations are inferences in the form of summary statements about the results of empirical or abstract theoretical investigations. In research, they involve a process of inferring general principles from particular pieces of evidence. For example, in experimental research the statistical analysis of the data might suggest that the findings are so strong that they are generalizable to other like cases that make up the larger population from which the study sample was drawn. Qualitative research findings resulting from intensive methods of content analysis also may suggest generalizations about the application of understandings derived from the study of one case to similar cases. A process of generalization is central to analysis within case as well. For example, in ethnographic research the strength of some evidence amassed is so consistent in descriptive detail that it suggests a cultural pattern into which subsequently obtained similar evidence will fit; that is, the pattern is inferred from the data.

Grand Theory

See **Broad-Range Theory** and **Model**.

Grounded Theory

Grounded theory method is a qualitative research approach developed by Glaser and Strauss (1967). It was a reaction against mainstream sociology's emphasis on (a) non-research based grand theory existing at a highly abstract conceptual level and (b) atheoretical research excessively focused on the technical aspects of quantitative methods. In an effort to bridge this perceived gap between theory and research, grounded theory emphasized the process of theory generation from systematically collected and analyzed data. The theory remains connected to ("grounded in") the data through descriptive examples from the research that show the fit between the theory and supporting empirical evidence. This close relationship with the data from which it was derived gives the theory much explanatory power. In turn, grounded theory can serve as a conceptual framework from which testable hypotheses may be constructed. Glaser and Strauss (1967) argued that verification of theory (hypothesis testing) was overemphasized in sociology, and consequently, caused qualitative theory-generating approaches to be undervalued. They viewed both theory development processes as mutually complementary and the associated research designs (theory testing/quantitative and theory generating/qualitative) as equal in status.

Grounded theory techniques for generating and analyzing data are similar to the field techniques of anthropological ethnographic method. Both rely heavily on skilled observation and intensive interviewing combined with systematic detailed record keeping and simultaneous processes of data collection and analysis. However, anthropological research focuses on cultural analyses and draws on a variety of theoretical perspectives. Grounded theorists focus on role development and role relationships from a symbolic interactionist point of view.

From the perspective of symbolic interaction, human behavior is the result of basic social processes. Individuals acquire a sense of self through interaction with others; and people, likewise, through shared experiences, create meaning that influences their collective behavior. That is, individuals as members of social groups align their self-interpretations with those of others and act in various situations according to those shared meanings and values. Research within this framework focuses both on the nature of social interactions and on the symbolic meaning conveyed by people's actions in varying circumstances.

Grounded theory involves a constant comparative method of analysis; that is, bits of data are continuously compared with other bits of data as they are acquired and over and over again across the life of the research. As data are compared for similarities and differences, they are coded; codes are compared and clustered to form categories of information; and categories are developed or collapsed into one another as a result of ongoing analysis. Memoing also occurs as a continuously flowing written record of ideas and hypotheses about the data. Data gathering is guided by an approach called theoretical sampling. The analysis of data suggests what further sampling is needed to develop categories or to validate or test hypotheses about the emerging theory. Thus, analysis directs sampling strategy and also sample size. When data collection ceases to produce new information, categories are established, and patterns in the data are clear, it may be presumed that closure, or saturation, has been achieved. Saturation of categories (sampling saturation) signals the end of data collection. However, an active search for negative cases, alternative cases that do not fit the pattern of the developing theory, may continue. Negative cases add depth and variation to the database and are important in verifying statements of relationship (hypotheses) derived from data analysis.

Process analysis is the main approach used to generate theory about social phenomena. The basic social process (BSP), or core category that is central to the theory, and/or related subcategories are usually gerunds (nouns ending in "ing"), indicating change in a process across time and variability according to conditions and circumstances. For example, Brown and Powell-Cope (1991) describe five subcategories of the core category "transitions through uncertainty," a substantive theory of AIDS family caregiving: (a) managing and being managed by the illness, (b) living with loss and dying, (c) renegotiating the relationship, (d) going public, and (e) containing the spread of HIV.

Approaches to grounded theory projects may differ. Stern (1994), who was mentored by Glaser, provides insights on the evolution of Glaserian and Straussian schools of grounded theory:

> Students of Glaser and Strauss in the 1960s and 1970s knew the two had quite different modus operandi, but Glaser only found out when Strauss and Corbin's *Basics of Qualitative Research* came out in 1990, whereupon Glaser wrote his second solo book on grounded theory, *Emergence vs. Forcing: Basics of Grounded Theory Analysis* (1992). (The first, *Theoretical Sensitivity*, was published in 1978.) (Stern, 1994, p. 212.)

Glaser (1992) claims that Strauss has departed from the original method of allowing the theory to emerge from the data, whereas Strauss points to how the method is being used and argues that change is inevitable, given the popularity and rapid diffusion of grounded theory approaches across research disciplines (Strauss & Corbin, 1994).

Reports of grounded theory research can be highly relevant and directly applicable to nursing practice in a wide variety of settings. As a qualitative method, its purpose is to generate theory that advances understanding of people's behavior in terms of underlying meaning and change in varying circumstances and over time. There are many examples of grounded theory research in the nursing literature. See, for example, Sohier's (1993) investigation of the grieving process in the parents of gay men dying from AIDS. Of particular interest is Morse and Johnson's (1991) collection of studies that may serve as examples of independent investigations of the illness experience, or taken together, may be used (as they are in the book) as the basis for a preliminary discussion of a formal theory of illness.

Also of interest is Wilson and Hutchinson's (1991) description of combining Heideggerian hermeneutics and grounded theory approaches as well as Beck's (1992, 1993) study of postpartum depression, using grounded theory and phenomenological methods on a single data set. Generally, mixing methods of research in a single study is considered to be risky business. Morse (1991b) states that "such mixing, while certainly do-able, violates the assumption of data collection techniques and methods of analysis of all the methods used" (p. 15). Stern (1994) also speaks critically about "muddling methods"; however, she adds that in cases where researchers choose to combine different qualitative methods, it is important to provide clear unambiguous information for readers on what they have done: " [Wilson and Hutchinson] . . . took great pains to tell us just what they did. . . . Beck let us in on what she had done. And that is the whole point, within the parameters of science: I really don't care what you do, just tell me about it. I might learn something" (p. 219).

For additional information on grounded theory method, see Glaser and Strauss (1967); Glaser (1978); Chenitz and Swanson (1986); Strauss and Corbin (1990, 1994); and Glaser (1992). For classical research examples, see Glaser and Strauss (1965), *Awareness of Dying*; Glaser and Strauss (1968), *Time for Dying*; Glaser and Strauss (1971), *Status Passage*; and Strauss and Glaser (1975), *Chronic Illness and the Quality of Life*.

G

75

Guttman Scale

A set of test items is said to constitute a Guttman scale if the response to any item is perfectly predictable from the total test score.

The term derives from the psychologist Louis Guttman (1941) who first developed the concept. Because no set of actual test items exactly satisfies the defining property, it is common to talk about the extent to which a collection of items does constitute a perfect Guttman scale. A statistic called the coefficient of reproducibility measures that.

Example: A test of racial prejudice consisting of items such as "I would be willing to vote for a person of another race," "I would be willing to marry a person of another race," and so forth should approximate a Guttman scale and have a very high coefficient of reproducibility. Respondents might "fall off the ladder" at different points of the scale, with some not even endorsing the former item, but anyone who endorses the latter item is almost certain to endorse the former item as well, so that there should be a very strong association between the *number* of items endorsed and *which* items are endorsed.

G

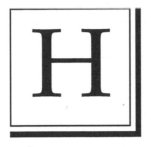

Halo Effect

Halo Effect is the name given to the phenomenon whereby people, such as evaluators, tend to be influenced by their previous judgments of something, such as performance or personality. The name implies that a good impression at the outset will carry over into future evaluations regardless of differences in quality or character of presentation. However, the same tendency would apply to an initial negative impression—that is, a negative bias similarly might carry over into future evaluations.

Halo Effect may be addressed by having evaluators complete an entire set of evaluations before moving on to the next and by concealing their previous responses as they move on to future evaluations.

See **Artifact**.

Hawthorne Effect

Hawthorne Effect is the name given to the phenomenon whereby people who know that they are participants in a study are likely to behave differently from the way they would behave without that knowledge.

The name comes from one of the original industrial-psychological studies, carried out in the 1920s at the Hawthorne plant of the Western

Electric Corporation in Cicero, Illinois. In that study no matter what sorts of experimental treatments were tried out on the employees (raising the lighting, lowering the lighting; raising the temperature, lowering the temperature; and other interventions) their productivity went up. The only explanation that could be provided at the time was that the employees were so grateful for the special attention that they tried to please the investigators in the best way they knew how, that is, by increased productivity.

The Hawthorne Effect can also work in reverse. People can be so upset about being studied that they perform *worse* than they otherwise might.

There are two "cures" for the Hawthorne Effect. The first, and better of the two, is to randomly assign experimental and control groups who *both* know that they are being studied; if the experimental group "wins" it will be an effect over and above the Hawthorne Effect. The second is to carry out research on human beings totally without their knowledge, so that the Hawthorne Effect has no opportunity to manifest itself. Such an approach raises some serious ethical problems, however.

Example: In an experimental study of the relative effects of visual stimuli and audial stimuli on reaction time, participating subjects should be told that they will be receiving one type of stimulus or the other, but they should not be told which one they will get. The Hawthorne Effect may operate, but it should be "balanced" across the two groups.

See **Artifact**.

Hermeneutics

The term "hermeneutics" derives from the Greek god, Hermes, who served the other gods as a bearer of messages to mortals. Historically, hermeneutic theory and method has been associated with the interpretation of Biblical texts. The original focus was on recovering the authentic versions of scriptures that were prone to numerous errors from hand copying prior to the age of the printing press. However, early in the 19th century, interest turned to issues of how to interpret any text not only by fixing attention on the work itself but also by taking into consideration the experiences of its author.

Reconstruction of the meanings that a writer has intended to convey implies a relationship between the reader and the text that is conversational in nature. For Wilhelm Dilthey (1833-1911), a German philosopher, the text expresses "lived experience" that can be understood by readers who try to put themselves in the position of the text's creator (an imaginative task made possible because of their shared humanity and the possibility of creating a spiritual bond). Similarly, other philosophers focus attention on the author's intended meanings and the importance of obtaining information about the writer of a text. For Gadamer, hermeneutic understanding involves creating a relationship between the linguistic and historical context of the interpreter and of the text to be interpreted and understood. This represents "the hermeneutic circle": the possibility of achieving understanding as the interpreter attempts to recapture the writer's perspective through dialogue with the text—asking questions of it, thoughtfully attentive for answers—effecting a partial bridging across time and space. An interpretation as rendered is never complete. It is always tentative, ongoing, and subject to revision in the hermeneutic circle.

Ricoeur extended the idea of hermeneutics as textual analysis to any human situation, which then is to be "read" as a text with attention to language and to silence—spoken and unspoken messages that reveal the substance of life experiences. The interpreter searches for the guiding metaphor that recaptures the meaning of a social situation. The emphasis of hermeneutics on understanding life through interpretation of human experiences is of interest to some qualitative researchers who look to place their work within a broad philosophical frame of reference. In turn, hermeneutics is at the core of projects within the humanities and sciences that are concerned with consciousness, symbolism, or spiritual aspects of people in social, cultural, or historical contexts and seek to express those concerns through interpretation of patterned or textual meanings.

For additional information, see Gadamer (1976), Ihde (1971), Palmer (1969), Rickman (1976), Ricoeur (1981), and Thompson (1982). See also Hiraki's (1992) critical hermeneutics study of the language used to describe, explain, and interpret the concept of nursing process in four introductory nursing textbooks.

Heuristic Research

Heuristic research is a style of qualitative analysis proposed by Moustakas (1967, 1990). It is similar to phenomenology in its focus on lived experience. However, Douglass and Moustakas (1985) point out some differences, including an emphasis on first-person accounts: "Whereas phenomenology loses the persons in the process of descriptive analysis, in heuristics the research participants remain visible in the examination of the data and continue to be portrayed as whole persons. Phenomenology ends with the essence of experience; heuristics retains the essence of the person in the experience"(p. 43, quoted in Moustakas, 1990, p. 39).

Major concepts and processes include (a) identifying with the focus of inquiry—open-ended, self-directed search and immersion in active experience; (b) self-dialogue—active dialogue with the phenomenon; (c) tacit knowing—comprehension; (d) intuition—bridging between implicit tacit knowledge and explicit knowledge that is observable and describable; (e) indwelling—developing reflective awareness of the meaning of the experience; (f) focusing—sustained and systematic process that produces insights; and (g) the internal frame of reference— depending on the internal frame of reference of the person who is having the experience (Moustakas, 1990, pp. 15-27).

See Lamendola and Newman (1994) for an example of a heuristic approach using Newman's method for pattern identification to examine the theory of health as expanding consciousness in persons with HIV/AIDS.

Hierarchical Regression

Hierarchical regression is a type of regression analysis in which the independent variables are "entered" sequentially into the analysis in accordance with some theoretical model. It tests the "effect" of one or more variables over and above other variables.

Reinhard (1994) used hierarchical regression analysis in a study of caregiver burden.

See **Regression Analysis**.

Historical Research

Historical research involves the systematic investigation and critical review of past events for the purposes of setting the record straight, discovering links with the past that explain or increase understanding of present events and circumstances, and answering questions about developments and trends.

> In contrast to nostalgia, history attempts to recapture the complex ways that the persons and ideas of the past have influenced the present. The understanding of history informs and shapes the view of contemporary life. Historical analysis of the past and the present is a subsidiary process that enhances our ability to criticize the decisions made in power realms that will certainly affect our future. (Hamilton, 1993, p. 48)

Historical inquiry involves intensive searches for, and concentrated analysis of, existing literature, documents, artifacts, photographs, and recordings on the subject of interest to the researcher. Oral histories, involving interviews with persons who are knowledgeable about historical events or personages, provide another type of information that broadens the range of data collection significantly. They allow for more creativity on the part of the researcher, who typically in historical research has no control over the quantity or the quality of data. With living sources of data, joint probing, searching, and reflecting on the targeted themes and questions may lead to rewarding and unexpected insights.

Sources of historical data are designated as primary sources (original documents, memorabilia, firsthand accounts) or as secondary sources (summaries and interpretations of primary source material by other persons). For example: "A nurse who served in the Anzio offensive during World War II is considered a primary source. In general, her observations about the experience will be more accurate than a secondary account of the same event provided by a daughter of another Anzio nurse who bases her story on information related by her mother" (Sarnecky, 1990, p. 5). Primary sources are of greater value because the potential for distortion or bias beyond the researcher's control is eliminated. Historical data are evaluated in terms of authenticity (external criticism) and estimated value or worth with regard to truth and accuracy (internal criticism).

The historiographer addresses research questions and/or tests hypotheses, sometimes statistically, but more often by logical interpretation of relationships among phenomena of interest suggested by the amassed data. Qualitative methods of data analysis may be used to arrive at inferences made by the researcher about hypothesized relationships. These involve identification of themes in the data content that will be analyzed and creation of categories to organize the data in meaningful ways and to enumerate or assess presence or absence of variables of interest. "By successfully combining science, art, and philosophy, history is three-dimensional. As a method or methods, it follows rules for ascertaining verifiable 'fact'; as synthesis and exposition, it calls for imagination, literary discrimination, and criticism; as interpretation of life, it requires philosopher's insights" (Cramer, 1992, p. 7).

Examples: Beeber (1990); Birnbach (1993); Bullough, Bullough, and Wu (1992); Bunting and Campbell (1990); Donahue (1985); Hughes

H

(1990); Norman and Elfried (1993); Norman (1992); S. Y. Stevens (1994); *Advances in Nursing Science* (1990, volume 12, number 4) issue on nursing history; *Nursing Research* (1992, volume 14, number 1) 40th anniversary issue.

Human Science

Human science is a term associated with a central theme of Wilhelm Dilthey's (1833-1911) philosophy of life, based on examination of human and social studies (*Geisteswissenschaften*). His interest was in the relationship between lived experience and understanding (*Verstehen*) of how the mind directs and reveals itself in history and literature. Today the term is used to describe a focus among a set of disciplines that includes anthropology, history, literary criticism, philosophy, psychology, and sociology, although the status of each in relation to this theme is continually in dispute. A human science focus is concerned with interpreting the meaning that various situations and life experiences have for people, in contrast to a natural science focus on providing causal explanations for them. The assumption is that nature can be explained, but humans need to be understood. Therefore, scientific methods must develop beyond experimental and test-related formulas for explanation to include interpretive approaches that generate understanding of human experiences. The latter approaches comprise the field of qualitative research.

Watson (1985) uses the notion of human science combined with human care to describe nursing. She asserts that a human science perspective is more consistent with nursing's historical focus on the whole person; involves a philosophical stance on human freedom, choice, and responsibility; and represents a moral tradition grounded in transpersonal caring, love, and connectedness. Watson (1985) exemplifies the distinction between human science and natural science approaches by contrasting nursing and medicine, and she uses the qualitative methods of phenomenology to develop her theory of human care:

> The goals for the theory ideals are associated with mental-spiritual growth for self and others, finding meaning in one's own existence and experiences, discovering inner power and control, and potentiating instances of transcendence and self-healing. . . . The context is humanitarian and metaphysical. It incorporates both the art and science of nursing. Science is emphasized in a human science context. . . . The

H

optimal method for studying the theory is more naturally through field study that is qualitative in design. (pp. 74, 76)

See **Phenomenology** and **Qualitative Research**.

Hypothesis

In the context of a scientific theory, a hypothesis is a statement that postulates some sort of a relationship between constructs (theoretical hypothesis) or between variables (operational hypothesis) acknowledged to be crucial to that theory. In the more restrictive context of inferential statistics, a hypothesis is a conjecture regarding the numerical value of a population parameter. The two meanings have a great deal in common, however, as inferential statistics often plays a central role in the testing of a scientific theory.

Example. "Infants born to heroin-addicted mothers have lower birth weights than infants of nonaddicted mothers" (Polit & Hungler, 1991, Table 8-1, p. 142).

Distinctions are typically drawn among hypotheses, propositions, axioms, and assumptions. Similarly, authors make distinctions among different kinds of hypotheses. For example, Polit and Hungler (1991) discuss deductive versus inductive hypotheses, multivariate versus univariate hypotheses, simple versus complex hypotheses, and so on.

In traditional statistical hypothesis-testing, a so-called "null" hypothesis is pitted against an "alternative" hypothesis. The null hypothesis is usually a conjecture regarding *no* relationship, *no* difference, etc., that the investigator is inclined to disbelieve; the alternative hypothesis is often a research hypothesis that arises from some theory that the investigator is inclined to believe. Sample data are collected and a decision is made to reject or to not reject the null hypothesis (one doesn't "prove" or "disprove" either hypothesis). The theory is thus strengthened, weakened, or modified.

The alternative hypothesis may be *directional* (e.g., the correlation between height and weight is greater than zero) or *nondirectional*, for example, the correlation between height and weight is not equal to zero. The first example postulates a directional difference from zero, whereas the second example is the simple denial of the null hypothesis.

Example: "Anxiety reduces achievement" is an example of an alternative research hypothesis that might be part of a theory of anxiety. To test that hypothesis one would actually determine whether or not its null counterpart, "There is no relationship between anxiety and achievement," can be rejected.

H

Hypothesis Testing

Hypothesis testing has both a general scientific meaning and a specific statistical meaning. Any study that tests one or more tenets of a theory is referred to as hypothesis testing. In addition, any study that employs a test of statistical significance is said to be using the hypothesis-testing form of statistical inference.

H

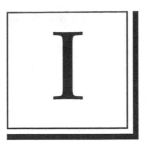

Idiographic Analysis

Idiographic analysis is concerned with the particulars or unique aspects of persons, events, or things. Generalizations are restricted to the specific case.

See **Case Study**.

Independent Observations

The observations ("pieces of data") in a research investigation are said to be independent if the measurement obtained on each subject neither influences nor is influenced by the measurement obtained on another subject.

The assumption of independent observations is crucial for all inferential statistical procedures but is often violated, especially in the application of chi-square to contingency tables. In such applications it is not uncommon to find that one or more persons has been counted in the data more than once. Whenever the number of observations is greater than the sample size there is a dependence-of-observations problem.

Example: In a study of the relationship between height and weight, Mary's height should be independent of Sally's height, unless they happen to be twins of one another. (Their weights are more likely to be more independent than their heights *even if* they are twins of one another.)

Independent Samples

Two or more samples are called independent if they are not matched with one another in any way.

Independent samples are very common in experiments; one sample is given the experimental treatment and the other sample is given the control treatment. They are also common in nonexperimental research concerned with sex differences, religious differences, and so forth.

Example: A cross-sectional study of the differences between 60-year-olds and 70-year-olds at a given point in time is likely to be based on independent samples (comparing a random sample of 200 60-year-olds with a random sample of 200 70-year-olds, say), whereas a longitudinal study of the differences between 60-year-olds and 70-year-olds must by definition use dependent samples (60-year-olds "matched" with themselves when they are 70-year-olds 10 years later).

Independent Variable

An independent variable is a variable that is a potential cause of a dependent variable.

In an experiment an independent variable is actually "manipulated"; that is, the investigator intervenes in the natural course of events and "creates" a variable of two or more treatment conditions. In nonexperimental research an independent variable is merely measured and correlated with a dependent variable.

Example: In testing the "effect" of stress on depression, where stress is the independent variable and depression is the dependent variable, one researcher might carry out an experiment by randomly assigning subjects to one of two stressful conditions and observing what happens to depression, but another researcher might measure stress, measure depression, and correlate the two.

Inductive Reasoning

Inductive reasoning is a way of thinking that is loosely described as moving from the specific to the general. In an emergent theory-building or research design, the process begins with the empirical observation. As description of phenomena in the observable world unfolds, ideas about how variables seem to be related are formed in the mind of the researcher. Generation of propositions, theory, or insights about the phenomena of interest comes through reflection on accumulating evidence, intuition, and introspection. The approach is most associated with qualitative research traditions. Induction is contrasted with deduction. However, both deductive and inductive modes of reasoning are applied to the analysis of data over time.

See **Deductive Reasoning** and **Theory**.

Inferential Statistics

Inferential statistics is the branch of statistics that is concerned with procedures for making generalizations from samples to populations.

Populations are usually very large and not completely accessible, and it is often too expensive to study *all* of the members of the population. Therefore, the researcher typically draws a sample from the population (ideally at random), studies the sample in *its* entirety, and makes some sort of generalization from the sample to the population. Such generalizations are always subject to error (the smaller the sample the greater the expected error) unless the population is perfectly homogeneous with respect to the variable(s) of concern.

If one happens to have data for an entire population, there is no statistical inference to be made, but some researchers choose to "regard" certain small populations as samples from larger populations (see Barhyte, Redman, & Neill, 1990).

Inferential statistical procedures are of two types: (a) those concerned with the estimation of population parameters and (b) those concerned with the testing of hypotheses about population parameters. The latter procedures are far more common.

Subsumed under estimation are point estimation, in which the researcher gives a "best guess" as to the actual value of a parameter, based on the calculated value for the corresponding sample statistic, and interval estimation, in which a "confidence interval" is established that has some specified probability of including the unknown value of the parameter. Point estimation is rarely employed, as it does not allow for any margin of error due to variability from sample to sample. Interval estimation is used quite often in survey research and in educational and psychological testing.

Rightly or wrongly, hypothesis testing gets "all of the play" in research conducted in most of the social and biological sciences (including nursing). There are two types of hypothesis-testing procedures: (a) parametric tests, which make certain assumptions about the population(s); and (b) nonparametric tests, which do not make such assumptions.

I

87

Example: If the average age of a random sample of 200 Alzheimer's patients is found to be 73.8 years, it might be inferred that the average age of the population from which that sample was drawn is 73.8 *plus or minus* 3 years. And the hypothesis that the average age of Alzheimer's patients is 80 would probably be rejected.

The foregoing remarks regarding the principal kinds of inferential statistics, as well as the distinction between descriptive statistics and inferential statistics, can be summarized as follows:

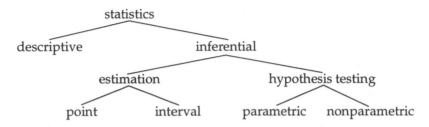

A particularly fine statistics textbook for nursing researchers is Munro and Page (1993).

Informatics

Informatics is a field of study that addresses the use of information technology. "Nursing informatics" is concerned with nurses' use of information systems in practice, administration, education, and research. Hays, Norris, Martin, and Androwich (1994) describe a number of milestones in the advancement of nursing informatics since 1970. Achievements include the evolution of client-centered record and information management systems, increased power and availability of technology, and organizational support for the ongoing development of nursing information systems.

The focus for the future is on next-generation nursing information systems. A report by the National Commission on Nursing Implementation Project (NCNIP) Task Force on Nursing Information Systems (Zielstorff, Hudgings, Grobe, & NCNIP, 1993) presents principles and guidelines for development of clinical systems in nursing practice, noting also the research commitment for nursing informatics studies.

Books on nursing informatics include Ball, Hannah, Gerdin-Jelger, and Peterson's (1988) volume on advanced concepts for experienced nurse informaticians and a primer for beginners by Hannah, Ball, and Edwards (1994). See also Sparks's (1993) article on electronic networking for nurses; Staggers and Mills's (1994) study of nurse-computer interaction, and *Advances in Nursing Science* (1990, volume 13, number 2) issue on nursing informatics.

See **Computer-Assisted Research**

Informed Consent

Informed consent is a term associated with research involving human subjects that is concerned with the extent to which the prospective participants are aware of the exact nature of the research and their right to agree or to decline to participate without fear of loss or reprisal. What they need to be informed *about* are such things as costs (e.g., physical and/or psychological risks) and benefits (e.g., personal compensation), how anonymity or confidentiality will be ensured, how the data will be collected and used, and their right to withdraw from the study at any time.

For obvious ethical and moral reasons, the privacy of research subjects should always be respected, and no person should be forced to participate in a study against his or her will. In response to a few rather flagrant violations of such principles by certain investigators, committees called institutional review boards (IRBs) have been mandated by law at virtually all major universities, hospitals, and other research institutions. These committees have been charged with protecting human subjects. Investigators who are planning to conduct studies that involve human beings directly must convince their committee that appropriate provisions have been made for informed consent before they are permitted to carry out the research. Signed consent forms are often obligatory.

Problems regarding informed consent are manifold, however. For example:

1. Who provides consent for babies? Or for the demented? And how about prisoners, students, and employees who are vulnerable to pressures to participate?
2. *How* informed must each subject be? Certain kinds of research are very hard to explain. Other kinds of research are pointless if the subjects are actually told the purpose of the research.
3. If "total" informed consent is not obtained beforehand, must the subjects be "debriefed" after the study has been completed? (In most cases the regulations insist that this be done.) If so, what form should debriefing take? Might some damage already have been done that is irreparable?
4. Does the filling out of an anonymous questionnaire constitute ipso facto informed consent? Can one always guarantee anonymity?

5. What happens when the IRB's concern for the protection of subjects' rights goes so far that entire study populations most in need of the help provided by research investigations become unavailable? (This is a particularly serious problem with many patients in nursing homes whose questionable ability to give true informed consent might result in their never being studied—see Robb, 1981.)

Instrumentation

Instrumentation is synonymous with measurement and is the term that is likely to be preferred in biophysiological research involving measuring devices actually constructed for some very specific purpose. The term is also preferred when identifying the data collection phase of the research design.

See **Design** and **Measurement**.

Intensive (In-Depth) Interviewing

Intensive (in-depth) interviewing involves a semistructured format and conversational style that allows the interviewer to probe for underlying emotions, thoughts, and meanings. It is a technique especially used in ethnographic and other qualitative approaches (e.g., grounded theory and phenomenologically oriented projects).

Interaction Effect

An interaction effect is a special kind of "combination" effect of two or more independent variables on a dependent variable.

It is an effect that is different from a simple summation of the effects of each of the independent variables taken separately. The term is usually associated with experimental research where a "sex-by-treatment interaction," for instance, may be of interest. The following example attests to other uses.

Example: If nurses have a life expectancy of 5 years above average, and researchers have a life expectancy of 3 years above average, one would expect that nurse researchers would have a life expectancy of 8 years above average. If they have a life expectancy either greater than or less than 8 years above average, then there is an interaction effect of the two independent variables (occupation and specialization) on the dependent variable (life expectancy).

Internal Consistency

Internal consistency is a type of reliability that is concerned with the extent to which the parts of an instrument "hang together." The most common procedures for determining the internal consistency of a measuring instrument are coefficient alpha (Cronbach's alpha) and split halves.

See **Coefficient Alpha**, **Reliability**, and **Split Halves**.

Internal Validity

Internal validity is a term that is synonymous with control. It was coined by Campbell and Stanley (1966).

A design (usually an experimental design) is said to be internally valid if the effect alleged to be produced by the independent variable can actually be attributed to that variable and not to some competing "threat" with which it is confounded.

As is the case with its companion term, external validity (generalizability), it is unfortunate that the term has the root word *validity*, because that is a measurement characteristic and not a design characteristic.

Example: A true experiment in which the subjects are randomly assigned to different drug treatments has very strong internal validity because the randomization process controls most variables that might otherwise be competing causes.

Interrater Reliability

Interrater reliability is a type of reliability that involves an assessment of the extent to which two raters (scorers, judges) agree regarding the ratings (scores, judgments) they give to the behaviors they observe. The term is synonymous with *objectivity*.

See **Reliability**.

Interval Estimation

Interval estimation is a type of statistical inference in which a "confidence interval" is constructed around an obtained sample statistic in such a manner that it has some specified probability of including the corresponding population parameter.

See **Inferential Statistics**.

Interval Scale

An interval scale is a level of scientific measurement characterized by the existence of a constant unit of measurement and an arbitrary zero point. The only permissible transformations of interval scales are those of the linear form $Y = a + bX$.

Example: Temperature measured on the centigrade (Celsius) scale is an interval scale, because the centigrade degree is constant throughout the scale, the zero point is arbitrary (the point at which water becomes ice), and the only permissible transformations are transformations such as the change from centigrade (C) to Fahrenheit (F) by the equation $F = 32 + 1.8C$.

See **Scale**.

Intervening Variable

An intervening variable is a variable that is in between an independent variable and a dependent variable in a causal sequence, and can therefore produce an *indirect* effect of the independent variable on the dependent variable in addition to, or instead of, a direct effect.

Example: Anxiety can have both a direct effect on achievement and an indirect effect on achievement through the intervening variable of (lack of) motivation.

Introspection

Introspection is an analytic technique used in qualitative research. It involves a process of recognizing and examining one's own inner state or feelings.

See **Qualitative Research**.

Intuition

Intuition is a sense of awareness or perception of meanings, truths, or feeling tones apart from any process of reasoning. Intuition and imagination are relied upon in qualitative analysis as a means of grasping or making sense of data.

See **Qualitative Research**.

I

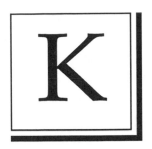

Key Informant

A key informant is a person who can provide detailed or specialized information about his or her own culture.

See **Ethnography**.

Known-Groups Technique

The known-groups technique is a procedure associated with criterion-related validity (some authors subsume it under construct validity). To "validate" a particular measuring instrument (e.g., a test of anxiety), an investigation is made of the extent to which a group of subjects known or assumed to possess a large amount of the trait being measured (e.g., anxiety) obtain scores on the instrument that are different from those obtained by a group of subjects known or assumed to possess a small amount of that trait.

An example of the use of the known-groups technique for instrument validation is provided by Janke (1994).

See **Validity**.

K

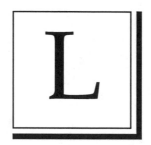

Law

A law is a proposition about the relationship between concepts in a theory that has been repeatedly validated and is confirmed. Laws are highly generalizable; that is, they are consistently supported and not tentative. The social/human sciences have few laws in comparison to the physical sciences.

See **Theory**.

Level of Significance

Level of significance, sometimes called significance level, is a term associated with the hypothesis-testing approach to statistical inference. It is the probability of rejecting a true null hypothesis, is usually denoted by the Greek letter alpha, and is conventionally set at .05, .01, or .001. For any given study, one and only one level of significance should be chosen, with all results interpreted with respect to that particular level (see Slakter, Wu, & Suzuki-Slakter, 1991).

See **Test of Significance**.

Life World/Lived Experience

In phenomenology, the life world (*Lebenswelt*), or lived experience, is the natural world in which humans live. Because it consists of the commonsensical and that which is taken for granted, it tends to be less accessible. The goal of phenomenology is to return to this familiar world and reexamine through reflective awareness what human experiences are like from that vantage point.

See **Phenomenology**.

Likert Scale

A Likert scale is a type of test item in which respondents indicate their attitude toward a particular statement by choosing one of a small number of ordered alternatives.

The term is derived from the industrial psychologist Rensis Likert (1932) who first used such scales. Most Likert scales consist of five scale points, usually designated by the words "strongly agree," "agree," "undecided," "disagree," and "strongly disagree." But there can be as few as 2 scale points or as many as 10 or more, and descriptors other than levels of agreement can also be used.

Example: In measuring attitudes toward abortion a researcher might present the statement "Abortion is murder" to a group of subjects and ask them to select one of the categories "yes," "under certain circumstances," or "no" that best expresses their feelings regarding that statement.

See **Scale**.

LISREL

LISREL is a computer program that is used to carry out structural equation modeling. It is generally favored by "East Coast" researchers in preference to EQS.

Johnson, Ratner, Bottorff, and Hayduk (1993) used LISREL to test Pender's Health Promotion Model.

See **EQS** and **Structural Equation Modeling**.

Logistic Regression

Logistic regression is a special type of regression analysis in which the dependent variable is a dichotomy.

For two articles regarding this type of regression analysis, see Yarandi (1993) and Yarandi and Simpson (1991).

See **Regression Analysis**.

Longitudinal Study

A longitudinal study is a type of research in which one or more groups of people is studied at several points in time.

L

Typical longitudinal research involves a single cohort (either an entire population or a sample therefrom) that is followed across time to investigate its development with respect to some dependent variable.

Example: A group of premature babies delivered at a particular hospital during a given calendar year might be followed up to determine if and when their weights "catch up" with those of full-term babies delivered in that same year.

L

M

Main Effect

Main effect is a term associated with the effect (causal or noncausal) on a dependent variable of a single independent variable considered separately from other independent variables.

The term is used most commonly in experimental research in which a factorial design assessing the effects of two or more independent variables has been used. The main effect of each independent variable is studied in conjunction with the combined (interaction) effects.

Example: The main effect of type of analgesic on reported pain is of considerable interest, in addition to the effect for males versus females, older people versus younger people, and the like.

Manipulation

Manipulation is the defining feature of an experiment. An investigation should be called an experiment if and only if the researcher directly "manipulates" the independent variable, that is, actively intervenes to create some sorts of treatment conditions.

Sometimes it is difficult to determine whether or not the manipulation criterion has been satisfied. If some person other than the researcher intervenes and the researcher then studies the phenomenon, a case could be made that such a study also falls under the heading of an experiment, even though the administration of the experimental treatments has not been directly under the researcher's control.

Example: An investigator who is sincerely interested in the effect of sex education on the incidence of teenage pregnancies should directly manipulate the independent variable by assigning students (ideally at random) to receive or not receive sex education, rather than seek out, after the fact, one group of students who have been exposed to sex education and another group of students who have not been exposed to sex education.

See **Experiment**.

Matching

Matching is a technique sometimes used in experimental research in which each subject receiving the treatment is paired with another subject not receiving the treatment in an attempt to control for one or more characteristics that the paired subjects have in common. It is often, but mistakenly, believed that such a technique is superior to random allocation of subjects to treatment groups. (Campbell & Stanley, 1966, discuss the weaknesses of matching as an experimental research strategy.)

See **Control** and **Blocking**.

Matrix (Matrices, pl.)

A matrix is an arrangement of data in rows and columns. Data may consist of numbers, as in a correlation matrix, or pieces of text that summarize research findings. Miles and Huberman (1984b, 1994) describe and discuss the use of matrices to facilitate three related subprocesses of qualitative data analysis:

1. Through *data reduction,* data volume is managed by sorting, summarization, coding, and clustering of information.
2. *Data display* of the organized, reduced set of data permits assessment of its completeness and provides a basis for drawing conclusions or taking action regarding needs for more information.
3. *Conclusion drawing and verification* involve interpretation of the data.

Use of matrices as part of an overall data management approach is aimed at keeping important data readily accessible, tracking data analysis, and retaining data and a record of the analysis beyond completion of the study.

See **Data Management**.

M

Mean

The mean (arithmetic mean) of a set of data for a variable is the sum of all of the scores (the term *score* is used to refer to any numerical measurement) divided by the number of scores. It is the most commonly encountered statistic in nursing research because it is the traditional "average" and researchers are often interested in the difference between the average scores on a particular variable for two or more groups of subjects, to determine the "effect" (not necessarily in the causal sense) of group membership on that variable.

Measurement

The term *measurement* is usually associated with the operationalization of abstract constructs into concrete variables but can include anything from careful description to formal assignment of numbers to objects according to well-defined rules.

When careful description is the main concern, there may be less conscious thought of operationalization. However, the fact that decisions must be made about which empirical realities to observe and how they will be observed implies some sort of operationalization.

It is helpful to think about measurement as the process of translating some sort of reality into numbers. When a construct, for example, height, is operationalized, each object to be measured is assigned a number. It may be very precise, for example, Mary is 68.7 inches tall; very rough, for example, Mary is a 1 (where 1 = tall, 0 = short, i.e., not tall); or anything in between.

The psychologist E. L. Thorndike (1918) once said: "Whatever exists at all exists in some amount" (p. 16). That claim was later followed up by the educator W. A. McCall (1939), who said: "Anything that exists in amount can be measured" (p. 18). To talk about something like height, sex, social support, or any other construct, it must be at least theoretically possible to measure it, and at least two different "scores" must be obtainable.

In quantitative studies measurement considerations arise when attention is given to data collection. This is sometimes called the "instrumentation" phase of the research, which comes between the overall design for the study and the analysis of the results. It is somewhat less important than the design phase, because unless the research problem is well thought out, good measures of various constructs won't help very much. But it is certainly much more important than the analysis phase, because meaningless measurements are not worth analyzing.

M

Example: The construct "Contraceptive Use" presents enormous measurement problems. First, is the focus to be on whether or not, which kind(s), how often, or just what? Second, how is the information to be obtained? Self-report? Probably, but such reports are subject to huge errors. Observation? Hardly, but that might be the most valid strategy. Third, who is (are) to be studied—only females who are involved in sexual activity? Only males? Both? If both, should *partners* be studied, given that contraception (or its lack) applies primarily to the act and not to the separate individuals?

By way of contrast, "Spelling Ability" poses far fewer problems. If you want to find out how much spelling ability a person has, you select a random sample of words from a dictionary and ask him or her to spell them.

Median

The median of a set of data for a variable is the middle value when the data are arranged from low to high (or high to low—it doesn't matter). The median is preferred to the mean when the variable being analyzed has a skewed frequency distribution and/or when the variable is ordinal rather than interval.

Mediating Variable

A mediating variable is the same as an intervening variable but usually carries the additional connotation of some sort of ameliorating or "buffering" effect.

See **Buffering Variable** and **Intervening Variable**.

Member Checks

In qualitative research, member checks involve ongoing informal and formal validation of data, analytic categories, interpretations, and conclusions with study participants from whom the data were collected. Member checking is a way of establishing the overall credibility of the research.

Memos/Memoing

In grounded theory and other qualitative research traditions, memoing, or the writing of analytical notes, is a part of the research process. It occurs across the life of the research and is a record of the ideas that the researcher has about the nature of the data and how different concepts may be linked to one another.

See **Grounded Theory** and **Qualitative Research**.

M

Meta-Analysis

A meta-analysis is a statistical amalgam of the findings of a number of research studies that have been carried out on a particular topic.

A meta-analysis is sometimes referred to as an "analysis of analyses" (Glass, 1976; O'Flynn, 1982), but it is really a *synthesis* (a bringing together of the analyses of separate investigations of the same general phenomenon) rather than an *analysis* (a breaking down). The original investigators have done the analyzing; the meta-analyst synthesizes the results of those analyses.

Although the term is somewhat grandiose (Glass, 1976)—and note that the prefix *meta* does not always carry the same meaning (Thomas, 1984)—meta-analysis is currently very popular, despite the contentions of a number of people (e.g., Eysenck, 1978) who argue that it is not a particularly worthwhile activity. Although it seems like an excellent idea to be able to quantify and integrate the findings of several studies, the technical problems are occasionally insurmountable.

There are a variety of ways of carrying out a meta-analysis. The most common way involves the determination of some sort of an average "effect size" across studies (again, see Glass, 1976). Most procedures make a number of difficult-to-defend assumptions, however, such as the independence of the studies and the comparability of the measurements for the study variables.

The term *meta-analysis* is sometimes confused with the term *secondary analysis* (for which this dictionary includes a separate entry). They are quite different activities. Glass's (1976) article makes the distinction very clearly and also points out how both activities differ from the "primary analysis" carried out by the original researcher(s).

Reynolds, Timmerman, Anderson, and Stevenson (1992) provide an excellent summary of meta-analysis and its advantages and disadvantages. For examples in nursing research, see Goode et al. (1991), Blegen (1993), and Krywanio (1994).

Metaparadigm

A metaparadigm represents the worldview of a discipline (the most global perspective that subsumes more specific views and approaches to the central concepts with which it is concerned). Nursing's metaparadigm generally is thought to consist of the central concepts of person, environment, health, and nursing.

See **Paradigm**.

M

Metatheory

Metatheory is a theory about theory and is concerned with generating knowledge and debate within a discipline around broad issues, such as the nature of theory in general, the types of theory needed by the discipline, and the suitable criteria for evaluating theory.

See **Theory.**

Method and Methodology

The terms *method* and *methodology* are often used interchangeably. For example, either term may be used as a section heading in a research report or as a chapter title in a dissertation. In that section or chapter the investigator describes in as much detail as space allows the design of the study and the actual procedures carried out in the collection and the analysis of the data. Here, method/methodology is to be contrasted with substance. The substance is the "meat" of the study—the concepts, the theory, the results, and so forth; the method is the "bones" on which the substantive findings are hung.

Overall, it would be useful to distinguish between method (set of techniques or procedures used to collect and analyze data) and methodology (study of the epistemological assumptions that guide the use of a method). Particular methods (techniques and procedures) may be common to a number of research approaches that differ importantly from one another in methodology. Stern (1994), for example, addresses this issue in noting that "muddling methods" in qualitative research is to be avoided: "Although there may be similarities in all interpretive methods, in that ethnographers, phenomenologists, and grounded theorists use observation and interview as a means of collecting data, the [methodological] frameworks underlying the methods differ" (p. 215). Morse (1991b) and Leininger (1994) also raise concerns about researchers who "mix methods" without sufficient understanding of methodological underpinnings.

Methodological Research

Methodological research is research on the tools of research. The focus of most methodological research is on the development of valid and reliable instruments that can later be used in substantive research. (A small amount of methodological research is concerned with issues of design and/or analysis.) There is a need in many kinds of nursing research to accurately measure cognitive and physical functioning or emotional responses of people. In some instances, instruments developed in other disciplines, for example, psychological profiles, life

M

satisfaction or quality of life inventories, and the like will serve the research purposes. In other instances, new or substantially revised instruments are created by investigators who want a scale, interview schedule, observational method, and so forth that will more specifically fit nursing practice. A disadvantage of creating instruments under circumstances that do not allow for much refinement of the methodology is the lack of adequate pilot testing and evaluation of the instrument, which in turn weakens conclusions drawn from the research as well as replicability. A pool of validated instruments that can be drawn upon by nurse researchers to measure different aspects of client response and nurse-client interaction in the contexts of illness care and health promotion is not yet available. Thus, methodological research is especially important in developing this type of resource.

For prototypical examples of methodological research in the nursing literature, see Nokes, Wheeler, and Kendrew (1994); Schraeder (1993); "Methodology Corner" in *Nursing Research;* "Focus on Psychometrics" in *Research in Nursing & Health;* and "Technical Notes" in *Western Journal of Nursing Research.*

Middle-Range Theory

Middle-range, or midrange, theory deals with some part of a discipline's concerns related to particular topics, for example, pain management, rehabilitation, or death and dying. The scope is narrower than that of broad-range or grand theories; that is, it is at a greater level of concreteness and specificity.

"Examples of middle-range theories in nursing include Orlando's (1961) theory of the deliberative nursing process, Peplau's (1952, 1992) theory of interpersonal relations, and Watson's (1985) theory of human caring" (Fawcett, 1995, p. 25).

See **Theory.**

Mode

The mode of a set of data for a variable is that value of the variable that occurs more often than any other value in the data.

Model

A model is a graphic or symbolic representation of a phenomenon that serves to objectify and present a certain perspective or point of view about its nature and/or function. Various media are employed in the construction of models, ranging from three-dimensional objects (such as plastic models of human organs and chemical structures

M

found in the biological and physical sciences) to diagrams, geometric forms, mathematical formulas, and words.

In nursing, a model is most often characterized as a *conceptual model,* a term that is used interchangeably with the term *conceptual framework.* The major nursing models identify concepts and describe their relationships to phenomena of central concern to the discipline: person/client, environment, health, and nursing. Examples include Johnson's model of the person/client as a behavioral system, Roy's adaptation model of person-environment interaction, Newman's model of health, and Orem's self-care model of client-nurse interaction. (See Fawcett, 1995; Fitzpatrick & Whall, 1989; and Marriner-Tomey, 1994.)

Many of the current nursing models are called grand theories (or simply, theories in the grand theory tradition) because of their global approach to the broad range of nursing practice. In discussions about differences between theories and models, most often the focus is on the precision with which concepts are linked with one another. Theories are thought to be more explicit than models in this regard.

Examples: King's (1971, 1981) conceptual model visualizes the world of nursing as being made up of dynamic open and interacting systems that she identifies as personal systems, interpersonal systems, and social systems. The relationships among these major concepts are elaborated in a general descriptive manner, and sets of concepts (subconcepts) associated with each system are further drawn out and defined in the second publication of her work. From this open systems model King has derived a theory of goal attainment that describes the sort of nurse-client interactions that lead to achievement of goals. She postulates that health/care goals that are mutually set by nurses and clients are attained through a continuing process of nurse-client actions, reactions, and interactions that results in transactions.

Another nursing model from which theory is being derived is Roy's (1984) adaptation model. The theory of the person as an adaptive system identifies four modes of adaptation (physiological, self-concept, role function, and interdependence) and attempts to explain how the relationships among concepts associated with each mode lead to adaptation.

Some authors suggest that it would be best to "minimize the differences between conceptual models, frameworks, and theories and to relegate most of these differences to semantics" (Meleis, 1991, p. 167). Others disagree, describing conceptual models as "general guides that must be specified further by relevant and logically congruent theories before action can occur" (Fawcett, 1995, p. 27). Lan-

M

caster and Lancaster (1992) assert that "substitution of one term for the other has led to their misuse":

> The position taken here is that all theories are models, because all theories purport to represent some aspect of real world phenomena. However, the converse is not true; all models are not theories because many models will not have all the requisites of theoretical construction. ... While a model describes the structure of events or systems, a theory moves beyond description to the level of prediction by stating relationships among components. (p. 434)

The greater precision and narrower scope of theories make them more amenable to testing; that is, hypotheses may be derived from the relational statements about concepts in a theory that may or may not be supported through research. Series of hypotheses have been generated by King and Roy in association with their theories. The partitioning of theories from more global conceptual models/frameworks results in consideration of sets of phenomena that are narrower in scope than their source, or middle range as opposed to grand phenomena.

Models that contain varying mixtures of scientific, philosophical, logical, and prescriptive dimensions provide guidelines for development of theory in certain directions in a discipline at the same time that they may restrict or limit development in other directions, especially if some models become dominant. Examples of well-known conceptual models (grand theories) that have influenced the generation of particular kinds of middle-range theories and related research in other fields are Einstein's theory of relativity and Freud's theory of psychoanalysis.

Conceptual models/frameworks in nursing tend to be pretheoretic models. That is, they represent preliminary theorizing, which serves heuristic purposes and provides a descriptive and philosophical base for later more formal theory building. However, models do not simply precede theory. In diagrammatic/schematic forms they may be used within a theory, serving as posttheoretic models to illustrate the structure of relationships or major features of the theory. At times the terms *conceptual model/framework* and *theoretical model/framework* are used interchangeably. Some authors encourage a distinction based on the pretheoretic bases of conceptual models/frameworks as opposed to the posttheoretic bases of theoretical models/frameworks—that is, theoretical models are constructed from theory and empirical research

M

findings, contain more specifically interrelated concepts, and are testable. Other authors consider conceptual models and theoretical models to be similar structurally, being composed of interrelated concepts that make up a whole, with theoretical models connoting "less tentativeness" than conceptual models (Chinn & Kramer, 1995, p. 219).

The terms *theoretical model/framework* and *theory* are also often used interchangeably. Again, some authors distinguish between models, in the schematic sense, which precede and coexist with theory, and theories, which provide fuller explanations of the phenomena in question.

Moderator Variable

A moderator variable is a variable consisting of two or more categories for which the relationship between two other variables differs from category to category.

The term is often used synonymously with *mediating variable* but should not be. (See Baron & Kenny, 1986; Lindley & Walker, 1993.)

Example: Sex might very well act as a moderator variable in the relationship between height and weight. For adult males the correlation between height and weight might be high and positive, whereas for adult females the correlation between height and weight might also be positive, but low.

Multicollinearity

Multicollinearity (some authors drop "multi") is a problem sometimes encountered in multiple regression analysis when the independent variables are very highly correlated with one another. In the extreme case, one of the independent variables may itself be a linear composite of two or more of the other independent variables, and this will make it impossible to actually carry out the analysis (the matrix of intercorrelations among the independent variables is said to be "singular").

Example: If Score on Part 1, Score on Part 2, and Total Score were all included as independent variables in a regression analysis there would be a multicollinearity problem because Total Score is equal to Score on Part 1 plus Score on Part 2 and therefore provides redundant information.

Multivariate Analysis

The term *multivariate analysis* usually applies to any statistical procedure that involves more than two variables. But some authors insist

M

that the term is appropriate only for analyses of multiple *dependent* variables, and they would not refer to multiple regression analysis (one dependent variable, any number of independent variables) or factor analysis (in which the independent vs. dependent distinction is not relevant) as multivariate.

To make matters even more confusing, hardly anyone calls "one-way" analysis of variance a multivariate procedure, as there is just one independent variable (often a "treatment" variable having several categories, or "levels") and one dependent variable (some sort of "response" or "criterion" variable in which the researcher is primarily interested). But if the independent variable has three or more categories, if these categories are "coded" into two or more "dummy" variables, and if multiple regression analysis (which is mathematically equivalent to the analysis of variance) is employed in the analysis of the data, there *are* more than two variables and the people who take the less restrictive view of the term should regard the analysis as multivariate.

The most common multivariate analyses are multivariate analysis of variance (one or more nominal independent variables and two or more interval dependent variables), discriminant analysis (just the opposite, i.e., two or more interval independent variables and one or more nominal dependent variables), and canonical correlation analysis (two or more independent variables and two or more dependent variables, all of which are usually of interval level). See Marascuilo and Levin (1983), Harris (1985), McLaughlin and Marascuilo (1990), or any other multivariate text for details.

Multivariate analysis is currently a fashionable buzz word. Researchers are thought to be really "with it" if they use some sort of multivariate analysis, because many variables impinge on a given problem. But it always has been, and always will be, "researcher's choice" regarding the number of variables she or he wants to study, just as long as they are relevant to the research questions. If a particular scientist chooses to study *only* obesity, say, or *only* the effect of the reduction in cigarette smoking *on* obesity, that scientist should feel free to do so and should resist pressures to include any additional variables.

Example: A defensible analysis of the research question "What is the effect of amount of salary increase on nurses' satisfaction and performance?" should consider satisfaction and performance in the *same* analysis, as they may be correlated with one another. It would be

M

inappropriate to undertake two analyses, one with salary increase as independent and satisfaction as dependent, and the other with salary increase as independent and performance as dependent.

M

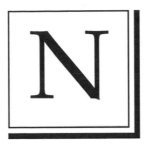

Narrow-Range Theory

Narrow-range, or micro, theory deals with a limited range of discrete phenomena that are specifically defined and are not expanded to include their link with the broad concerns of a discipline, for example, explanation of physiological or psychological phenomena.

See **Theory**.

Need Analysis

Need analysis uses the problem-solving process and is a type of applied research similar to evaluation research. Its purpose is to collect, organize, and present information that describes problems or needs of a target population and evaluates their importance and relevance in comparison to wants and demands (McKillip, 1987).

Need analyses are undertaken by agencies and service organizations for a variety of reasons: in connection with decisions to expand services, write proposals to obtain program funding, adapt to changing needs of consumers, attract additional types of clients, set budget priorities, or implement new procedures. Basic steps of the process include (a) describing the target population and the service environment; (b) identifying needs by describing the type and extent of problems, expressed needs, expected outcomes of what could or

N

should be, and the impact, cost, and feasibility of solutions; (c) assessing the importance of the needs by judging if the current or proposed programs or services satisfy people's wants (i.e., they will be utilized) and meet a demand (i.e., there is a market based on expressed needs of consumers); and (d) communicating results in the form of written or oral reports, tables, graphs, and figures.

Different need assessment models may focus on (a) expert opinions and values (discrepancy model—examines differences between what ought to be and what is); (b) values and concerns of consumers (marketing model—develops a competitive marketing mix to maximize utilization by the target population); and (c) values of decision makers who will use the results of the need analysis (decision-making model—provides an index that orders options on need across attributes or results of measures and information gathered for the need analysis). (See McKillip, 1987, pp. 19-31 for fuller description and examples of models.) Multiple methods for data collection and analysis are often used: inventories, surveys, statistical measures, social indicators, cost analysis, utilization analysis, and interviews with groups and key informants.

See **Applied Research, Problem Solving,** and **Evaluation Research.**

Negative Cases

In grounded theory, a negative case is an exception or variation—a case that does not fit into existing categories or support statements of relationships (hypotheses). Searching for negative cases produces variation in the data that serves to deepen understanding and extend the evolving theory.

Drummond, Wiebe, and Elliott (1994) present data analysis of a negative case that was used to validate a theory about maternal understanding of infant crying.

Negative Relationship

A negative relationship between two variables, say X and Y, is one in which Y increases as X decreases and Y decreases as X increases. It is also called an inverse relationship.

If the Pearson product-moment correlation coefficient is used to measure the relationship between two variables, a negative relationship is indicated by a number between -1 and 0.

A common confusion is to think of a negative relationship as *no* relationship (because of the word "negative"). A negative relationship

N

of −.70 is actually a stronger relationship than a positive relationship of +.50.

Example: There is a negative relationship between bowling scores and golf scores; that is, as golf scores go down bowling scores tend to go up. Note, however, that this is simply an artifact of how the two games are scored. The two *traits,* bowling ability and golf ability, are actually positively related. The reader is cautioned to be on the lookout for that same sort of phenomenon when interpreting negative correlation coefficients that are reported in nursing research.

Nominal Scale

A nominal scale is a level of scientific measurement consisting of a set of unordered categories. Any numbers can be used as labels for the categories.

Example: Religious affiliation is a typical nominal scale. Each person being "measured" for religious affiliation is given a number that is a label for a category (e.g., Protestant = 2), but the numbers have no other numerical interpretation.

See **Scale**.

Nomothetic Analysis

Nomothetic analysis is concerned with finding general laws that subsume individual cases. It involves generalizing from one case to a larger group of which it is thought to be representative, or comparing the single case with another group in order to identify the differences.

See **Case Study**.

Nonparametric Statistics

Nonparametric statistics are inferential statistical procedures that do not make any assumptions about the shape of the population distribution and do not place any restrictions on its parameters.

They are to be contrasted with parametric statistics such as the "pooled" *t* test of the significance of the difference between the means of two independent samples, which assumes that the corresponding populations have normal distributions and equal variances.

There are two common misconceptions regarding nonparametric statistics. The first is that they are to be used for small samples. The second is that they are descriptive rather than inferential statistics. These confusions may result from the understanding that for small samples it is inappropriate to use the sample variances and the normal sampling distribution to test differences between means (the sample variances might provide poor estimates of the population variances) and because of the close association between certain descriptive statistics, such as Spearman's rank correlation coefficient or Kendall's tau, with nonparametric inference.

The principal sourcebook for nonparametric techniques is Siegel and Castellan (1988).

Example: One of the most popular nonparametric statistics is the Mann-Whitney U Test for two independent samples in which the differences between ranks are examined rather than the differences between actual scores.

Nonrecursive Model

In path analysis and structural equation modeling a nonrecursive model is one in which some of the causal relationships are postulated to be reciprocal.

See **Path Analysis** and **Structural Equation Modeling**.

Null Hypothesis

A null hypothesis is a specific conjecture regarding the value of a population parameter that is usually postulated for the express purpose of being rejected by the sample data.

There are two reasons for the modifier "null": (a) the hope that the hypothesis gets "nullified" by the data and (b) the fact that most null hypotheses claim that some parameter is equal to zero.

Example: There is no relationship between age and pulse rate.

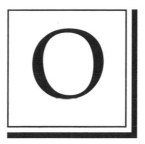

Observation

The term *observation* is used in two different senses in nursing theory and research. One meaning is as a procedure for gathering data that requires the investigator to witness and record certain behaviors. The other meaning is as a piece of data, as in "The total number of observations for this study was 73."

In the former sense of the term, the modifiers "participant" and "nonparticipant" are sometimes used to indicate the level of involvement of the investigator in the study environment.

In the latter sense, an observation may be "univariate" or "multivariate"; that is, it may be a measurement taken on a single variable or a set of measurements taken on several variables. In any statistical analysis it is essential that the observations be independent—that there is a one-to-one correspondence between subject and observation. It is very common for researchers to collect data in such a way that some subjects are counted in the data once, others are counted twice, still others are counted five or more times, and so forth. That creates havoc with many tests of statistical significance, such as the chi-square test, for which one of the assumptions is the independence of the observations.

O

Example: Obstetric nurses interested in the behavior of mothers when feeding their newborn babies might unobtrusively observe such behavior and record the number of smiles or hugs, whether or not or for how long a time the mother "coos" to the child, and so forth. The resulting data then become the observations that can be subjected to one or more statistical analyses. Thus in the same study the word "observation" could be used in both of its senses.

One-Tailed Test
A one-tailed test is a test of statistical significance in which the null hypothesis is pitted against a directional alternative hypothesis.
See **Alternative Hypothesis, Null Hypothesis**, and **Test of Significance**.

Ontology
Ontology is a branch of metaphysical inquiry in philosophy that is concerned with the study of existence itself and the nature of reality. Theoretical perspectives and approaches to research are influenced by ontological assumptions about the nature of reality. For example, natural science approaches involve a view of reality as reducible to separate variables and processes, any of which can be studied apart from others. Human science approaches assume reality is a composite of multiple inseparable realities that are irreducible and can only be studied holistically.

Operational Definition
Operational definitions link theoretical constructs with the real world by identifying what phenomena (empirical indicators/referents) will be observed and how they will be measured. Concrete ideas (e.g., weight, blood pressure, touch, activities of daily living, fluid intake) are not too difficult to operationalize because empirical indicators can be specified with some precision and direct measurements may be made. However, research concerns in nursing frequently involve abstract notions (e.g., social support, self-esteem, adaptation, sensory deprivation, body image, health, or well-being) that do not have exact empirical indicators and can only be measured indirectly. Complex and abstract constructs have many aspects. Operationalization thus becomes a process of sorting out aspects and choosing which one(s) to feature in the research. Brink and Wood (1983) demonstrate how one such abstraction, anxiety, can be defined or conceptualized

in different ways. Each conceptualization of anxiety suggests a different measurement approach:

1. "Vague feelings of alarm that persons report when faced with a stressful situation" (involving self-report as measurement)
2. "Behavioral manifestations of persons subjected to stress, which can be identified by grimaces, muscle tensing, and palmar sweating" (involving observation)
3. "A trait possessed by all persons to some degree, which is reflected in their responses to questions about their view of life in general" (requiring "that the researcher infer how the individual feels from his or her responses to questions.") (p. 75)

The authors conclude, "None of these is a perfect measure; none is better than the others" (Brink & Wood, 1983, p. 75).

The investigator is free to choose one method or multiple methods of measurement. Even so, the process of operationalization in a single piece of research will often limit to some extent the number of ways in which variables may be explored. The least limiting approaches to operationalization involve qualitative methods aimed at producing rich description. Such methods involve a very broad range of observations and measurement styles. Thus, they often do not involve narrow operational definitions that would preclude description of the different ways in which the variables of interest manifest themselves. Other types of research require a more restricted focus, which means that the researcher must choose to feature some aspects and ignore or downplay others.

It is not unusual for other people to question or disagree with the way in which investigators have operationalized constructs. Nevertheless, a benefit of a precise operational definition lies in its ability to clearly communicate the researcher's perception of, for example, anxiety, within the context of the particular research. The implications of research results are also clearer when examined in the light of this established framework. No delimited set of operational definitions or single piece of research can account for the complexity of some constructs. Careful operationalization of constructs, however, can help to provide meaningful insights on which further research may build.

Oral History

Oral history captures original thoughts and meanings that are woven into spoken accounts of personal experiences. Historians, biographers, and social scientists may collect oral histories as a way to preserve valuable primary data as well as to understand and represent the historical and cultural realities that are revealed in these narratives. Oral communication research strategies can be used effectively to capture oral traditions, to increase understanding by reducing cultural gaps between researchers and participants, and to make it possible for the "voices" of marginalized groups and individuals to be heard.

Unstructured interviewing techniques generally are used to provide breadth and allow individuals to tell their stories in their own ways. See Paterson and Bramadat (1992) for discussion of the use of the preinterview in oral history. Audio or video recording often is used.

An example of oral history in nursing is the pioneering project involving interviews of six nursing leaders who helped to advance the mission of the New York State Nurses' Association (NYSNA). A collection of videotapes and a publication including six monographs, transcripts, biographical data sheets, and references are available from the NYSNA library (Carter & Fielding for NYSNA Council on Nursing Research & the Foundation of NYSNA, 1988). See also Yow's (1994) guide for recording oral history.

See **Historical Research** and **Biographical Method**.

Ordinal Scale

An ordinal scale is a level of scientific measurement consisting of a set of ordered categories. The numbers used as labels for the categories signify relative order but not quantity. The numbers can be transformed into any other numbers that are in the same order as the original numbers (e.g., 2, 3, 4, 5, 7 are just as appropriate as 1, 2, 3, 4, 5).

Example: A typical ordinal scale is a Likert scale with the categories strongly agree, agree, undecided, disagree, and strongly disagree.

See **Likert Scale** and **Scale**.

Orthogonal Design/Rotation/Contrasts

The term *orthogonal* is used in at least three different senses in research, all of which have the general connotation of independent or unrelated.

An orthogonal design is a balanced design in which all main effects and all interaction effects can be assessed independently of one another.

An orthogonal rotation in factor analysis is a transformation of factor loadings in such a way that the underlying factors remain uncorrelated with one another.

Orthogonal contrasts are comparisons carried out in the analysis of variance such that the result of one comparison has no influence on the result of another comparison. For example, a contrast of Christians versus Jews and a contrast of Catholics versus Protestants are orthogonal because the second contrast involves the comparisons of two religions on "opposite sides of the ledger" that were on "the same side of the ledger" in the first contrast.

Outlier

An outlier is a data point that appears to be isolated from the other data points and may therefore be the result of an unusual measurement error.

It is very common in scientific research to employ some sort of procedure to try to identify outliers and to correct them or delete them from the data analysis. The reason is that even a single outlier can have a profound effect on the determination of a mean, a standard deviation, a correlation coefficient, or any of a number of statistics that may be used to summarize the research findings, particularly if the sample size is small.

Example: If measurements of the number of children in ten families yield the values 0, 0, 1, 2, 2, 2, 3, 3, 5, and 22, the 22 should be carefully checked to see if a reporting or recording error might have been made (perhaps it should have been 2 but that digit was inadvertently repeated?). Otherwise the results could be quite distorted. With the outlier the mean would be 4; without it the mean would be 2. The differences in the standard deviations in the two cases would be even more pronounced, and if that variable were to be correlated with a variable for which the 22 were paired with another outlying value, that single data point could "anchor" the correlation coefficient at an artificially high level.

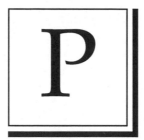

Paradigm

The term *paradigm* is sometimes used interchangeably with the term *model*. However, it is more customary to think of a paradigm as a larger organizing framework that contains:

1. Concepts, theories, assumptions, beliefs, values, and principles that form a way for a discipline to interpret the subject matter with which it is concerned
2. Research methods considered to be best suited to generating knowledge within this frame of reference
3. What is open to investigation—priorities and views on knowledge-deficit areas where research and theory building is most needed
4. What is closed to inquiry for a time

A paradigm is similar to an action plan that describes work to be done in a discipline and frames an orientation within which the work will be accomplished. Examples of paradigms that have guided theory building and research in other disciplines include evolutionism, structuralism, functionalism, economic determinism, and the psycho-analytic approach. Meleis (1991) observed that nursing has been heavily influenced by paradigms from other fields, for example,

118

psychoanalysis; developmental, adaptation, and interaction theories; and humanism.

A discipline may have a number of specific paradigms (exemplar paradigms) that direct scientific work. Typically, there will be disagreement over which is "the best" for explaining phenomena of concern. A type of paradigm called a metaparadigm, however, subsumes different more specific paradigms to create, at a more abstract level, a worldview for the discipline that takes in what the phenomena of concern are. This does not rule out a variety of perspectives and methods that provide different views of metaparadigm concepts. There is general agreement that nursing's metaparadigm consists of the central concepts of person, environment, health, and nursing (Fawcett, 1995).

Nurses who cite Kuhn (1970, 1977) have described nursing as being at a "preparadigm" stage of development (i.e., where there is lack of agreement about a paradigm that contains requisite information on central concerns and how to study them). Kuhn's (1970) revolutionary theory of scientific development describes a progression in disciplines from prevailing paradigm, to dispute, crisis, and revolution over that paradigm. The outcome is the establishment of a new prevailing paradigm around which members of the field are unified. The periods of calm between crises are called "normal science"—that is, one paradigm dominates and alternatives are not accepted.

Kuhn has had both followers and critics. Lauden (1977) in particular has remarked on the rigidity of Kuhn's theory and its inability to account for real-life activities of development and testing of theory that continually act in a corrective way to bring paradigms ("research traditions") into question, adjust them, and extend them. Not only do disciplines maintain a variety of coexisting traditions, but "Many of the theories within an evolving research tradition will be mutually inconsistent rivals, precisely because some theories represent attempts, within the framework of the traditions, to improve and connect with their predecessors" (Lauden, 1977, pp. 81-82).

Meleis (1991) suggests that nursing knowledge has not developed through a revolutionary process as described by Kuhn. She proposes "integration" as the pattern of progress in nursing that accounts for accommodation of multiple paradigms and tolerance of theoretical pluralism in the discipline:

> A case for paradigmatic pluralism has to be made in nursing because there is a need for theories about people, interactions, illness, health, and

nursing interventions. In fact, currently there are many different theories that, although seen by some as competing with each other, address different relationships and focus on different phenomena, thereby actually complementing each other. These theories evolved from a variety of paradigms (adaptation, system, and interactionist, among others). (Meleis, 1991, p. 79)

Parallel Forms

The parallel forms technique is a method for assessing the reliability of a measuring instrument that has two or more interchangeable operationalizations.

See **Reliability**.

Parameter

In statistics, the term *parameter* has one and only one meaning, and that is as a descriptive index of a population (a population mean, a population standard deviation, a population correlation coefficient, etc.). Population parameters are constants that are usually unknown but are hypothesized about or estimated from sample data.

The term causes a great deal of difficulty because in mathematics a parameter is not a constant but a variable (x is a function of t, y is a function of t, and the like), and some researchers use the term in a similar sense to refer to a dimension that is of direct concern in the problem that is being investigated (e.g., "The parameters we are interested in are sex, age, height, and weight").

In more general parlance a parameter is some sort of boundary condition ("Within what parameters are we permitted to operate?"). That meaning derives primarily from confusion with the word *perimeter*, however.

Another context in which the term *parameter* arises is in computer programming. In that context a parameter is a piece of information that needs to be specified for the software to execute a command.

It is the statistical meaning that is most commonly encountered in nursing research.

Example: An interesting, but unknown, parameter is the percentage of American nurses who smoke cigarettes. It has been estimated in a number of studies (see, e.g., Wagner, 1985) but no one really knows how small or how large that percentage actually is.

Partial Correlation Coefficient

A partial correlation coefficient is a special type of correlation coefficient that indicates the magnitude and direction of the relationship between two variables with one or more other variables statistically controlled ("partialed out"). It is to be contrasted with a zero-order correlation coefficient, which does not involve any "partialing." If one variable has been statistically controlled, the coefficient is called a first-order partial coefficient; if two variables have been statistically controlled, the coefficient is called a second-order partial coefficient; and so forth.

There is also such a thing as a semipartial correlation coefficient, which, as the name implies, involves statistical control with respect to one of the two variables but not the other.

Partial correlations were used by Walker and Montgomery (1994) in their study of maternal identity and role attainment.

See **Zero-Order Correlation Coefficient**.

Participant Observation

Participant observation is the central technique used in anthropological fieldwork. It involves direct observation of everyday life in study participants' natural settings and participation in their lifeways and activities to the greatest extent possible.

Participant observation results in copious fieldnotes. Adequacy of fieldnotes rests on how extensive and inclusive they are and on the quality of descriptive detail, that is, their ability to reconstruct situations covering all the actors involved, including the researcher; sensitivity to language differences, what people actually say, and how they express themselves; attention to people's appearance, actions, and nonverbal cues; and use of introspection to assess the researcher's opinions, impressions, and possible influence in the situation.

See **Ethnography**.

Path Analysis

Path analysis is a special application of regression analysis. Prior to the actual carrying out of the regression analysis the researcher displays in a pictorial model (called a path diagram) the kinds of causal relationships that are alleged to hold. The regression analysis then provides some evidence regarding the plausibility of the model. It does not demonstrate that such causal relationships actually exist; it strengthens or weakens the *case* for causality.

P

P

The associated vocabulary for path analysis differs somewhat from the vocabulary of traditional regression analysis. Instead of independent and dependent variables one speaks of exogenous and endogenous variables. The former are those variables whose causes are not under investigation; the latter are those whose direct and indirect causes are of concern within the model. The magnitudes of the effects of the exogenous variables upon the endogenous variables, and of some of the endogenous variables upon other endogenous variables, are called path coefficients (they are actually partial regression coefficients—standardized or unstandardized). Models that postulate only one-way causation are called recursive; those that allow for reciprocal causation are called nonrecursive.

There are additional technical terms for specific aspects of path analysis, such as the matters of "identification" and "specification" (see Pedhazur, 1982, for details).

Example: A path analysis might be carried out to determine the direct effect of stress on depression and the indirect effect of stress on depression as mediated by social support. Such a model is an integral part of many theories regarding the relationships among those variables (e.g., Norbeck, 1981) and can be diagrammed as follows:

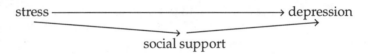

For more complicated, but more realistic, examples of path analyses in nursing research, see Smyth and Yarandi (1992) and Lucas, Atwood, and Hagaman (1993).

Pearson Product-Moment Correlation Coefficient ("Pearson *r*")

The Pearson product-moment correlation coefficient, affectionately known as Pearson *r*, is a statistic invented by the British statistician Karl Pearson for summarizing the magnitude and the direction of the linear relationship between two variables. It can take on any value between −1 (perfect inverse relationship) and +1 (perfect direct relationship).

Percentage

As is well known, a percentage is a number that indicates part of a whole. It can take on any value between 0 (none) and 100 (all). Percentages over 100 are occasionally encountered in statements such as "The average salary for beginning staff nurses has increased by over 200% in the last three decades," but references to percentages greater than 100 are rarely found in nursing research reports.

Phenomenology

Phenomenology is a way of thinking about what life experiences are like for people. In philosophy, it refers to a method of inquiry developed by Edmund Husserl (1859-1938). Husserl followed the desire of his teacher Franz Brentano (1838-1917) to reform philosophy by developing it into a rigorous science given over to serve the best interests of humanity. For Husserl, this involved a critique of positivistic science as abstract and incapable of dealing with human experience because of its refusal to consider anything other than observable entities and objective reality as a focus of study. Husserl argued for a return to "the things themselves," essences that constitute the pre-scientific world of human consciousness and perception. He introduced the concept of the life world (*Lebenswelt*), or lived experience, as the natural world in which we live. However, the life world is not readily accessible because it is made up of what we take for granted and therefore fail to explore. Husserl believed that the logic of what is taken for granted—all that is commonsensical, unsophisticated, and naive—is the foundation and source upon which objective (positivistic) science draws. The task of phenomenology is to return to the familiar and reexamine what we believe we already know and understand by reflectively bringing into awareness what has been taken for granted. Phenomenological research always asks about the nature or meaning of the human experience—What is it like?

The question is answered by means of a process of phenomenological reduction. It involves studying various types of data that describe the experience (e.g., interview data, written narratives, letters, diaries, literature, art) and engaging in a largely introspective sort of communication with those data. Introspection is accompanied by continuous writing and rewriting as an interpretation of meaning develops and becomes increasingly refined. The goal of phenomenological writing is to heighten critical awareness and deepen reflective thoughtfulness about what is important in the taken-for-granted and seemingly trivial aspects of everyday life.

There are different schools of thought within phenomenology and well-known personalities who have become identified with particular interests and styles. Researchers may claim to base their work on views regarding fundamental issues and approaches (e.g., Husserlian

P

phenomenology, Heideggerian phenomenology). Research labels may also reflect a particular mode within which the writer is working (e.g., existential phenomenology, transcendental phenomenology, hermeneutic phenomenology). Phenomenological sociology has generated various perspectives that share a common intellectual base in the work of Husserl and Alfred Schutz. Schutz's work of applying principles of philosophical phenomenology to sociological questions is complex and has been subject to conflicting interpretations. Consequently, there remain within sociology approaches that are phenomenological only in a very loose sense—that is, the only thing they share with phenomenology is a concern about the importance of subjective meaning in the interpretation of social behavior. Another type of phenomenological sociology is reflected in the work of Berger and Luckmann (1967), who tried to blend the focus of phenomenology on individual consciousness and subjective meaning with sociological concerns about social structure on a larger scale (a phenomenology of the social world). It has been argued that yet another area of sociological practice, ethnomethodology, combines phenomenology and sociology to produce a uniquely different type of inquiry.

Cohen and Omery (1994) describe the characteristics of three phenomenological traditions most used in social science research: (a) eidetic (descriptive) phenomenology, in the tradition of Husserl or the Duquesne school (Giorgi, Colaizzi, Fischer, and vanKaam); (b) interpretive phenomenology, in the tradition of Heidegger or Heideggerian hermeneutics; and (c) some combination of descriptive/interpretive goals, in the tradition of the Dutch phenomenology of the Utrecht school (Barritt et al. and van Manen).

It is unlikely that there will be a single unified approach to thinking about and doing phenomenology. The unifying thread in phenomenological research is exploring what people's lived experience is like; and individual researchers are obliged to explain the theoretical perspective that guides their work and the methods they use to produce an interpretation of lived experience from their data.

Phenomenological writing is essentially a solitary effort requiring patience and practice, and it is dependent upon literary skill and creativity. Some general notions of what is involved are common to most descriptions of the method. One is bracketing, in which one identifies and tries to hold in suspension whatever beliefs and opinions one might have acquired in life about the phenomenon. Another involves retention (remembering and keeping in mind the details of described experience); reflection (going over and over details, viewing the experience from different perspectives, and trying to capture its most salient features along with the feeling of it); and imagination (free associating—trying to recall similar experiences in one's own life and what they were like). Finally, an interpretive grasp of what the meaning or feeling tone of the experience may be completes the reduction process. It requires imagination and intuition, first, to imagine different types of life circumstances to which one's awareness of what the experience was like might apply; and second, to transmit through writing the feeling tone derived from the experience that may be generalized to a broader field of human experience. For example, a few lines from van Manen's (1986) book *The Tone of Teaching* express a feeling tone that can transcend the boundaries of teacher-student situations and be equally recognizable as something that humans experience in other kinds of situations:

How Do Children Experience Our Presence?

We may be physically present to children while something essential is absent in our presence. Similarly, we may be physically absent from children while in a different sense they remain present in our lives after school, and we remain present to them. This happens to a child doing homework who feels the teacher looking over his or her shoulder. Or to a teacher preoccupied with something that happened during the day who cannot put a particular child out of mind. (p. 43)

To bring into awareness what has been taken for granted suggests that reader response to the above passage could be: we have all had the same kind of experience; we recognize the feelings the text draws out; it brings back memories.

There is no one particular way of structuring a phenomenological interpretation; van Manen (1990) suggests some possible ways to organize the account—thematically, analytically, exemplificatively, existentially, and exegetically. The extent to which the writing captures feeling tone is less dependent on organization, as it is more of a matter of rigorously writing and rewriting until the language finally expresses the feeling of the experience in a thoughtful and sensitive way. See, for example, Olson's (1993) work, *The Life of Illness*, illustrating phenomenological writing that uses personal experience, dialogues, and excerpts from literature describing the experience of illness.

Phenomenological research does not generate empirically based descriptions or theory. It is a qualitative investigation that provides descriptive/interpretive accounts of the body, space, time, and human relations as they are lived. Its humanistic focus can be characterized as a type of ethical activity in that its aims are (a) to explore and redefine what is possible within the realm of various human experiences, and (b) to evoke a thoughtful response with regard to what ought to be. As such it offers an alternative to objective, rationalistic methods of evaluation.

Other readings (philosophy and psychology): Heidegger (1962, 1975), Husserl (1965, 1970, 1977), Ihde (1971), Jaspers (1968), Merleau-Ponty (1962, 1964), Natanson (1973), Reeder (1986), Spiegelberg (1982), and Stapleton (1983).

Other readings (nursing): Benner (1994), Criddle (1993), Diekelmann (1992), Drew (1993), Jacobson (1994), Kondora (1993), Lauterbach (1993), Munhall (1994), Porter (1994), Rather (1992), Ray (1994), and Tanner, Benner, Chesla, and Gordon (1993).

Philosophical Research

Philosophical inquiry in nursing has been described as "virtually unexplored territory" and as yet "in its infancy" (Kikuchi & Simmons, 1992, pp. vii, 105). In contrast to scientific inquiry, it is the most abstract, and it is discursive rather than investigative in nature. Its purpose is to answer questions that do not lend themselves to scientific study: "Scientific questions . . . are questions regarding the phenomenal (material) aspects of reality. . . . When we are faced with philosophical questions (speculative questions regarding metaphysical aspects of reality and the normative questions grounded in them), science's investigative observational and measurement tools are useless" (Kikuchi, 1992, pp. 28, 29-30).

There are several types of philosophical questions: (a) ethical questions such as what ought to be, how one should be, what is good, and what principles apply in various types of situations; (b) epistemological questions dealing with the nature of knowledge and what counts as knowledge; and (c) ontological, metaphysical questions concerning existence itself, or being.

Fry (1992) observes that although everyone asks philosophical questions and can participate in argumentation, "extended philosophical investigation requires more than everyday knowledge about philosophy" (p. 88). Thus, there is a historical and continuing tendency within nursing to engage in philosophical discussions, particularly around ethical concerns or epistemological issues, such as the nature and scope of nursing knowledge. However, often there is incomplete appreciation of the basic philosophical nature of questions and failure to recognize the characteristics of work that is essentially philosophical in approach. Overall, there is a need for sustained dialogue about the scope and methods of formal philosophizing and for a substantive literature base (beyond extant examples of critical analytic, phenomenological, and hermeneutic work that address limited aspects of the philosophical enterprise).

Kikuchi and Simmons (1992) summarize a number of issues that need to be addressed before the potential of philosophical inquiry in nursing can be fully actualized, including (a) Is there to be a unifying theme for philosophical investigations, or is diversity of thought to be preferred? (b) Can unity and diversity of thought coexist in nursing? (c) What role will philosophical inquiry occupy in the discipline in terms of unique contributions and in relation to scientific and contemporary conceptualizations of nursing? (d) What conditions are required for the development and support of philosophical inquiry in nursing? and (e) Who has the responsibility for answering nursing's philosophical questions, and on what basis should that be decided? Although the future of philosophical inquiry in nursing remains unclear, there is evidence of investment in this type of work on the part of a small community of scholars. Fry (1992) reflects that: "In the final analysis, perhaps it is not philosophical inquiry that has been neglected in nursing scholarship, but rather our openness to visualize philosophical inquiry as necessary and fundamentally important with respect to establishing the theoretical foundations of nursing practice and research" (p. 94). Certainly, questions about vision and the mission of scholarly practice in this area will need to be resolved at the interface of philosophical and scientific inquiry where differences and convergence will be most apparent (Simmons, 1992).

Pilot Study

A pilot study is a preliminary trial of a research project with a small group of subjects who are similar to those to be recruited later. The purpose is to allow the researcher and any assistants to practice and evaluate the effectiveness of proposed data-collection and analysis techniques. Thus, problems with the methods can be detected and changes made when necessary before the large-scale project is launched. In addition, unexpected responses and findings may suggest new directions for the investigation or point out discrepancies that may need to be addressed.

Small-scale exploratory investigations are sometimes called pilot studies even though a larger study is not specifically planned at the time when they are undertaken. This may reflect the preliminary nature of the work, a need for baseline data, or the intention of the researcher to build research on the database generated by the pilot study. Many student theses, because of limitations of time and resources, could be identified as this sort of study.

The important thing when a pilot study precedes a planned study is to perform every step as it will be performed in the projected research. The main interest of the investigator is usually in the adequacy of data-collection instruments. "Pretesting" of instruments and "pilot studies" are sometimes discussed together in research texts as separate but related concepts. Pilot studies are more comprehensive, incorporating pretesting data-collection instruments along with a trial run of a study on a smaller scale that includes data analysis and reporting results.

For additional information on pilot studies, see Prescott and Soeken (1989). For an example of a pilot study, see Barkman and Lunse (1994).

Placebo

Placebo is a general term for a treatment that is very similar to the experimental treatment except that it lacks the essential ingredient that is of principal interest to the researcher.

The term comes from medical research, specifically from research on the effects of drugs such as aspirin or other analgesics. To pin down the effect of certain drugs it is essential to have at least two groups of subjects; the experimental group gets the pill (or liquid, or whatever) with the drug and the placebo group gets the pill (or liquid, or whatever) without the drug.

Example: If a researcher in nursing education wanted to test the effect of a particular film on the attitudes of nursing students toward abortion, she or he might randomly assign the students to two groups; one group would view the abortion film and the other group would view a film with similar content but without any reference to abortion per se.

Point Estimation

Point estimation is a type of statistical inference in which a single sample statistic is claimed to be in some sense the "best" estimate of the corresponding population parameter.

See **Inferential Statistics**.

Population

A population is an entire set of people or hospitals or whatever is of particular interest to the researcher.

See **Inferential Statistics**, **Parameter**, and **Sampling**.

Positive Relationship

A positive relationship between two variables, say X and Y, is one in which Y increases as X increases and Y decreases as X decreases, although not necessarily in perfect lockstep order. It is also called a direct relationship, but that term has a slightly different meaning in certain contexts such as path analysis in which the distinction is made between direct and indirect rather than between direct and inverse.

When the Pearson product-moment correlation coefficient is used to measure the relationship between two variables, a positive relationship is indicated by a number between 0 and +1.

Example: There is a positive relationship between height and weight for adult American females; that is, taller women tend to be heavier and shorter women tend to be lighter, but there are many exceptions. The Pearson r is approximately +.50.

Posttest

In experimental research a posttest is a test that is administered after the experimental manipulation has taken place.

See **Experiment**.

Power

In a test of statistical significance, power is the probability of not making a Type II error, that is, the probability of correctly rejecting the null hypothesis when it is false.

See **Test of Significance**.

Predictive Validity

Predictive validity is a type of criterion-related validity in which the data for the external criterion are obtained after the data for the instrument to be validated have been gathered.

See **Validity**.

Premise

A premise is an introductory propositional statement about the relationship between concepts in a theory. In deductive logic, prem-

P

ises serve as the basis for forming a conclusion. Postulates and axioms are other types of premises.

See **Theory**.

Pretest

In experimental research a pretest is a test administered before the experiment is undertaken.

See **Experiment**.

Primary Source

A primary source is a source of original data, such as documents, memorabilia, or firsthand accounts. Primary sources are preferred over secondary sources because of the decreased potential for bias and distortion beyond the control of the researcher.

See **Secondary Source**.

Probability Sampling

Probability sampling is a type of sampling in which each object in the population has a known (but not necessarily equal) probability of being selected into the sample.

See **Sampling**.

Problem Solving

Problem solving is a process that uses research methods to meet program needs and to solve concrete problems. It tends to be cyclic in nature, involving assessment of a situation, setting goals and implementing a plan, evaluating the effectiveness of the plan, and making revisions, at which point the cycle repeats itself.

See **Evaluation Research**, **Need Analysis**, and **Research**.

Process Analysis

Process analysis is the central analytic approach used in producing grounded theory. It is concerned with change in social phenomena over time, integrating stages or phases that people go through, and identifying supporting processes and modifying conditions.

See **Grounded Theory**.

Proportion

Like a percentage, a proportion is a number that indicates part of a whole. It can take on any value between 0 (none) and 1 (all), it can be easily converted to a percentage by multiplying by 100 and affixing a

% sign, and it is usually preferred for summarizing part/whole evidence in most statistical work.

Example: If a sample contains two males and three females, the proportion of females is 3 out of 5, or .60; the percentage of females is $.60 \times 100 = 60\%$.

See **Percentage**.

Proposition

A proposition is a statement about the relationships between concepts in a theory. It is a general label that includes postulates, premises, axioms, theorems, hypotheses, and laws. The terminology for different types of propositional statements varies according to the contexts in which they are used and the formal purposes served in logical deductive reasoning formats.

See **Theory**.

Prospective Study

A prospective study is a type of correlational research in which two or more groups of subjects are followed across time and compared on one or more variables.

Williams, Oberst, and Bjorklund (1994) report the results of a prospective study of women with hip fractures.

See **Correlational Research**.

Protocol

The term *protocol* refers to the overall plan or "recipe" for procedures to be carried out in a particular study. The term is frequently used by biophysiological researchers and is concerned with exclusion criteria, the specific regimen to be followed, and the like.

Purposive Sampling

Purposive sampling is a type of nonprobability sampling in which the researcher selects for study only those subjects that satisfy prespecified characteristics.

P

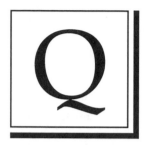

Q Sort

A *Q* sort is a measurement strategy first introduced by the psychologist William Stephenson (1953) as a self-report technique for determining the relative relevance to an individual subject of a set of declarative statements. The subject is given a deck of cards, one statement per card, and is asked to sort those cards into several piles with designations ranging from "most like me" to "least like me." The number of piles and the number of cards to be placed in each pile (but not which cards) are predetermined by the researcher and usually chosen so as to form a normal or near-normal frequency distribution.

Example: A nursing researcher interested in the reasons why people select nursing as a profession could prepare cards listing 16 reasons that might be given and ask each prospective student nurse to sort a deck of cards containing those reasons into five piles, with one card to be placed in the first pile (the subject's most compelling reason), four in the second pile, six in the third pile, four in the fourth pile, and one in the last pile (the least compelling reason).

For an example of a nursing research study that used a *Q* sort, see Puntillo and Weiss (1994).

Qualitative Research

Qualitative research is a cover term for a variety of research traditions originating in philosophy, anthropology, psychology, and sociology that are epistemologically and methodologically similar in many respects, although they differ distinctly in others. Epistemology is concerned with how people come to know the world in which they live. A qualitative perspective reflects one side of a debate in modern philosophy between a realist and an idealist view of the world. Realism asserts that physical reality exists independently of being perceived. Realist philosophy is associated with "the received view" of what is to count as knowledge. The label, applied by Putnam (1962), reflects a history of domination for over 30 years by 20th-century scientists who espoused recognition of only one investigative approach, "the" scientific method. From the realist, or received-view perspective, the purpose of research is to describe, explain, and predict subsequent occurrences of objectifiable phenomena in order to produce or control desired outcomes. In contrast, idealist philosophy questions the possibility of a mind-independent world, insisting that the external material world is known through the perceptions and subjectivity of humans. This constitutes a qualitative perspective, associated with "the nonreceived view" in the philosophy of science. The purposes of the various types of qualitative research involve description and interpretation of human experience in ways that promote understanding, provide insight, or challenge existing beliefs about, or perceptions of, social situations and human experience. Many qualitative researchers consider the above differences in epistemological assumptions about ways of knowing and understanding phenomena to be the main distinction between quantitative and qualitative methods of research.

Methodological similarities across qualitative traditions extend to techniques of data collection and analysis that include:

1. Personal involvement with informants in their natural settings
2. Intensive (in-depth) interviewing and detailed description of observations and conversations
3. Self-reflection and introspection to bring forward one's own inner feelings and intuitive responses to the data
4. Openness to discovery of the unexpected
5. Willingness to redirect the research as new insights and understandings emerge from the simultaneous process of data collection and data analysis

6. Management of often-large volumes of descriptive data through various approaches to content analysis that may involve coding the data (e.g., by number, color, word label) to break it down into some form in which it can be manipulated, organized and examined more easily; grouping similar data into categories; memoing, or writing analytic notes to keep track of ideas that the researcher has about the nature of the data and about how different concepts may be linked to one another; and reflectively reading and rereading, writing and rewriting, interpretations of meaning or feeling tones inherent in the data

Because data collection and data analysis occur simultaneously throughout the research, with analysis driving subsequent approaches to sampling and data gathering, researchers often work toward saturation. Theoretical saturation is a sense of closure that occurs when data collection ceases to provide new information and when patterns in the data become evident. Personal saturation is the sense of completion experienced when the researcher concludes that the aims of the analysis have been carried out as far as possible.

It is important to emphasize again that qualitative research is not one method but many; and a focus on commonly employed techniques of qualitative researchers is an insufficient and misleading orientation to this diverse field. Despite similarities, qualitative traditions differ in history, substance (major assumptions, major concepts, shared understandings, orientation, and purpose), and preferred methods. Anthropological methods, such as ethnography, and qualitative approaches in sociology, such as grounded theory, were first introduced to nursing by nurses who obtained doctoral degrees in those disciplines. More recently, phenomenology and other approaches to philosophical analyses also have been introduced. The first nursing texts specifically addressing qualitative research were published in 1985 and 1986 (Chenitz & Swanson, 1986; Field & Morse, 1985; Leininger, 1985; Munhall & Oiler, 1986; and Parse, Coyne, & Smith, 1985). From that time, reported research and discussion of qualitative research methodologies have been increasing. The popularity of qualitative research, however, raises concerns about (a) adequacy and appropriateness of mentoring for students and support for researchers and (b) availability of forums for dialogue about maintaining standards and resolving methodological issues. Morse's (1991c, 1994) companion volumes on contemporary "sticky" and critical issues in qualitative research (in nursing and across disciplines) are excellent sources of information about questions and needs

134

to be addressed in coming years. (See also Morse's editorials and the section called "Pearls, Piths, and Provocation" in *Qualitative Health Research* for an ongoing overview of ideas and concerns in this field.)

The growth of qualitative research, in general, has reflected several trends: (a) rising interest in human science approaches across many academic and practice fields; (b) a convergence of social science disciplines in recent years in which there is increased regard for the philosophical bases of research, greater tolerance for multiple research approaches, less specialization and distinctiveness in terms of methodology, and more interdependence in research focus, analysis, and application; and (c) greater appropriation of social science approaches to research by researchers in applied fields, with or without appreciation for and attention to the context within which those approaches are grounded. There is continuing need for (a) prototypical examples of research conducted within the frameworks of known traditions, (b) careful examination of how distinct traditions within qualitative research may be used in complementary ways in a single investigation, and (c) ideas that address the issue of how to label research purported to be "qualitative" by virtue of techniques employed but lacking the substance that would evidence grounding or fit within a recognizable qualitative research tradition.

The appropriateness of combining qualitative and quantitative approaches in a single research project continues to be debated. Historically, those who believe that the differences between quantitative and qualitative research approaches are primarily technical (different data collection and analysis techniques) have advocated "mixing and matching" methods to fit the needs of the research question (Goodwin & Goodwin, 1984). Those who believe the differences to be primarily epistemological (different ways of knowing about phenomena) have asserted that "one cannot mix methods across qualitative and quantitative paradigms . . . [because] mixing methods, goals and purposes across the paradigms violates the intent and philosophic purposes for each paradigm" (Leininger, 1994, p. 101). In response to Goodwin and Goodwin's (1984) position, Powers (1987) stated that techniques are subordinate to a larger theoretical stance:

> How data are managed reflects the paradigm within which they are produced. For instance, qualitative data can be used in a quantitative research design . . . [and] quantification can be part of a qualitative design. . . . There is no problem with subordinating certain techniques

> to others in performing research in either the quantitative or the qualitative tradition . . . [but] in single studies that use qualitative and quantitative data sets, the paramount concern must be with stating or uncovering the dominant paradigm that guides the research. (pp. 125-126)

Morse's (1991a) discussion of ways to implement qualitative-quantitative methodological triangulation also rests on the stated assumption that "the first step is to determine if the research problem is primarily qualitative or quantitative" (p. 120).

Rigor is of concern both in quantitative, hypothetico-deductive studies and in qualitatively designed investigations. All research needs to be subjected to evaluative criteria that are most appropriate for determining its soundness. In measurement studies, the reliability and the validity of the instruments and the data-collection procedures are the appropriate criteria. In qualitative studies, accuracy and credibility are frequently used criteria, and there are a variety of descriptors that amplify what those concepts mean when applied to an evaluation of the "goodness" of a qualitative design or product. Some qualitative researchers use terms that parallel the concepts of reliability and validity (e.g., Lincoln & Guba, 1985; Miles & Huberman, 1984a; Sandelowski, 1986). Others question the wisdom of mirroring the criteria of research modes that differ so much from qualitative products. Leininger (1994) has identified and defined six criteria to use in evaluating qualitative studies: (a) credibility, (b) confirmability, (c) meaning-in-context, (d) recurrent patterning, (e) saturation, and (f) transferability. In addition, Sandelowski (1993, 1994) has revisited her earlier discussion of "rigor" in qualitative research, emphasizing the importance of balancing scientific rigor and the "artfulness" of the qualitative craft: "What seems clearer to me now . . . and what I hope to clarify here, is that rigor is less about adherence to the letter of rules and procedures than it is about fidelity to the spirit of qualitative work" (1993, p. 2).

Rigorous and well-conducted qualitative projects can provide empirically based conceptualizations of phenomena, theories, and theoretical frameworks that give a sound basis for narrower theory-testing types of work. Nursing has become increasingly aware of theory building and the importance of theory-linked research. Theory-generating research typically employs a qualitative perspective and involves an inductive approach focused on discovery and description of experience and observed real world events.

In addition to the generative power of qualitative research in the domain of theory construction, qualitative studies may also reveal aspects of human and social behavior (e.g., complex personal relationships, subjective responses, perceptions) that cannot be tapped by other research methods. Important insights that could increase the understanding of people's needs in relation to health care situations are often missed or misperceived because they are buried in ordinary situations that are relegated to the category of "common sense" or "what everybody already knows." Qualitative research projects tend to focus on what is commonplace, take nothing for granted, and search for underlying meanings with the potential to refocus and redirect nursing practice by sensitizing research consumers, provoking people to a higher level of thoughtfulness, or challenging and questioning what is taken for granted--confronting and working to change the status quo. Qualitative research is descriptive to some end; that end in any of the qualitative traditions often has been of a reactionary or reformatory nature, to transform as well as to inform.

See **Quantitative Research.**

Quality Assurance
See **Evaluation Research.**

Quantitative Research

Although the term is not explicitly used very often, quantitative research is concerned with precise measurement, replicability, prediction, and control. It includes techniques and procedures such as standardized tests, random sampling and/or assignment, tests of statistical significance, and causal modeling. It may be preceded by descriptive pilot studies that are preliminary steps to a subsequent experimental or correlational study.

Quantitative studies have one or more of the following properties:

1. Adoption of the hypothesize-test-rehypothesize sequence that is characteristic of "the" scientific method
2. Emphasis upon structured and objective measuring procedures
3. Extensive use of numbers to reflect the measurements and to summarize the results
4. An emphasis on causality

Path analysis, treated elsewhere in this dictionary, is a prototypically quantitative research approach. A model regarding one possible state of the world is postulated, tested, and (if warranted) revised. Data for testing the model are usually based on objective measuring instruments. The numbers yielded by those instruments are analyzed to produce other numbers that assist the researcher in deciding which hypotheses in the model to accept and which to reject.

The label of quantitative research is not a good one, though, because it is difficult to call to mind any study that does not or could not involve some quantification. When quantitative research is contrasted with qualitative research (an equally problematic cover term), the label has come to stand for an orientation characterized by the insistence that science can only deal with observable phenomena and that systemically controlled and regulated observation and experiment will reveal general laws that demonstrate the relationships between phenomena. The orientation comes from a belief that the social and human sciences can be scientific in the same way as mathematics or physics, and thus, there is a distinct preference for measurement and quantification, as well as a tendency to deduce explanations of social phenomena that avoid focusing on or dealing with human subjectivity—perceptions, intentions, motives.

It is more accurate to regard differences between quantitative and qualitative research as differences in research purpose and orientation than it is to differentiate between such studies on the basis of preferred methods, for example, whether they involve description or quantification. Quantitative approaches have descriptive aspects and qualitative approaches may use counts, measurement techniques, and statistical analyses. The techniques are not the basis for the ways in which research is labeled. The purpose and nature of the investigation best reveals the sort of orientation being taken, as follows:

Quantitative research: Hypothetico-deductive in nature with the aim to test, predict, and control

Qualitative research: Interpretive and inductive in nature with the aim to generate theory, insight, and understanding

See **Qualitative Research**.

Quasi-Experiment

A quasi-experiment is an experiment that has manipulation and some controls but lacks random assignment of individual subjects to the treatment conditions.

True experiments with random assignment are thought to provide the most powerful tests of research hypotheses concerned with cause-and-effect relationships, because of the extent to which extraneous influences may be controlled. There are many instances, however, when a true experiment is not feasible, that is, random assignment cannot be carried out. For such quasi-experiments serious consideration must be given to other factors that might possibly have affected the outcome of the study. These alternative explanations are called "threats to internal validity." Quasi-experimental designs attempt to compensate for the absence of randomization in various ways. (See Campbell & Stanley, 1966, and Cook & Campbell, 1979, for descriptions of a number of quasi-experimental designs.) In spite of their limitations, quasi-experiments are frequently more practical in nursing research that takes place in settings less amenable to full experimental control.

Some authors (e.g., Polit & Hungler, 1991) define a quasi-experiment as an experiment that involves any two out of the three features (manipulation, control, randomization) of a true experiment. Other authors use the term quasi-experiment very broadly to denote any "experiment-like" study that involves the comparison of two or more groups, with or without the actual manipulation of the principal independent variable by the researcher.

Example: Since it is at best awkward to randomly assign individual Alzheimer's patients to receive Drug A or Drug B, the investigator interested in determining the relative effectiveness of the two drugs might choose to give Drug A to patients in one health care facility and to give Drug B to patients in another health care facility, and use some sort of statistical procedure such as the analysis of covariance to adjust the data to take into account the fact that the groups may not have been equivalent at the beginning of the experiment. Note, however, that any sort of statistical control is inferior to the direct control provided by the random assignment that is characteristic of a true experiment.

Quota Sampling

Quota sampling is a type of nonprobability sampling in which, as the term implies, sampling continues until certain quotas are filled. It is used quite frequently in certain kinds of opinion polls that attempt to sample so many women, so many men, so many Whites, so many Blacks, and so forth. The typical pollster may be asked to walk down a city block and find a Black female, a male over 35 years of age, and so forth.

Quota sampling should not be confused with stratified random sampling, which is a type of probability sampling.

See **Sampling**.

Q

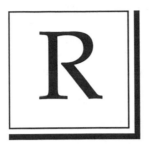

Random Assignment

Random assignment is a means of control in a true experiment. Individual subjects are allocated to the treatment conditions in such a way that chance and chance alone determines which subjects receive which treatments.

Groups to which subjects are randomly assigned may be judged to be equal in a statistical sense at the beginning of the experiment, although they may not actually be equal in every respect. As the sizes of the groups increase, so does the probability that they are similar, if random assignment has been carried out properly.

Random assignment may be accomplished by using coins, cards, tables of random numbers, or other devices that eliminate any biases that an investigator may have, consciously or unconsciously, in allocating subjects to treatment conditions.

Example: A nurse physiologist carrying out basic research on rat endocrinology might randomly assign half of a sample of rats to receive an injection of one type of hormone and the other half to receive an injection of a second type of hormone in order to study the comparative effects of the two types of hormones on feeding behavior.

Random Sampling

Random sampling is a type of sampling in which chance and chance alone determines which subjects in a population are drawn into a research sample. The purpose of random sampling is to provide a statistical basis for generalizing the results of the research from the sample actually employed to the larger population of interest.

Simple random sampling is a type of random sampling in which every subject in the population has an *equal* chance of being drawn into the sample. *Stratified* random sampling necessitates the division of the population into two or more subpopulations called strata and taking a simple random sample from each stratum.

Just as for random assignment, devices such as coins, cards, or a table of random numbers can be used to draw the sample. But it is essential to keep in mind that random sampling and random assignment are *not* the same thing.

The terms *random sampling* and *probability sampling* are often used interchangeably.

Example: In attempting to estimate the percentage of registered nurses who smoke cigarettes, a researcher might obtain a directory of all registered nurses in a particular state and use a table of random numbers to select the sample to whom a self-report questionnaire could be mailed.

Randomized Clinical Trial

A randomized clinical trial is a true experiment characterized by manipulation of the principal independent variable, random assignment of individual subjects to the treatment conditions, and any additional controls thought to be necessary. There are a number of synonyms for this term, such as randomized trial, controlled clinical trial, and true experiment.

Such experiments are used quite frequently in drug research and are often "double blind" to prevent additional biases that might be attributable to knowledge by the experimenters or the subjects of treatment membership.

Example: A nurse researcher who is interested in studying the effects of presurgical information on postsurgical recovery might design an experiment in such a way that patients are given various printed descriptions of things to expect, with the specific information to be given to each patient randomly determined and coded so that the "level" of information being transmitted is blind to the patient and to the distributor of the information, and known only to the investigator.

For an example of an actual randomized clinical trial in nursing research, see O'Sullivan and Jacobsen (1992).

Range
The range of a set of data for a variable is the difference between the lowest value and the highest value for the variable.

Ratio Scale
A ratio scale is a level of scientific measurement characterized by the existence of a unit of measurement and a "real" zero point that is indicative of absence of the construct being measured. The only permissible transformations of ratio scales are those of the restricted linear form $Y = bX$.

Example: Force (in dynes, say) is a typical example of a ratio scale. A "score" of zero on that variable means no force. There is nothing special about the dyne, however; any multiplicative transformation to some other convenient unit is perfectly acceptable.

See **Scale**.

Recursive Model
In path analysis and structural equation modeling a recursive model is one that admits only one-way (i.e., not reciprocal) causation.

See **Path Analysis** and **Structural Equation Modeling**.

Reduction, Phenomenological
Phenomenological reduction is an introspective process that produces expressions of what life experiences are like for people. It involves bracketing, retention, reflection, imagination, and intuition that lead to an interpretive grasp of what the meaning or feeling tone of the experience may be.

See **Phenomenology**.

Reflection
In phenomenological research, reflection involves mentally reviewing and going over and over the details of the lived experience under study, viewing it from different perspectives, and trying to capture meaning and feeling tone.

See **Phenomenology**.

Regression Analysis
Regression analysis is a statistical procedure for studying the relationships between variables and determining the extent to which

143

independent variables, individually and collectively, can predict and/or explain some dependent variable.

The focus of the regression analysis may be any or all of the following:

1. The determination of a mathematical model that best fits the data. This model is in the form of a linear regression equation, $Y = a + b_1 X_1 + b_2 X_2 + \ldots + b_p X_p$, where Y is the dependent variable, the Xs are the independent variables, a is the intercept, the bs are the regression slopes, and p is the number of independent variables.
2. The determination of how well the model fits the data.
3. The determination of the statistical significance of the fit.

Those who emphasize the regression equation itself are concerned primarily with the regression coefficients—the intercept (a) and the slopes (the bs). (The slope is equal to zero and the bs are called beta weights if the regression equation is in standardized form.) Those who concentrate on how well the equation fits the data emphasize correlation coefficients or their squares, which give some indication of the extent to which the independent and dependent variables vary together. Those who pursue the statistical significance of the intercept, the slopes, the squares of the correlation coefficients, and so forth are attempting to ascertain whether or not the fit of the equation to sample data could be attributable to chance alone.

There are several types of regression analyses: simultaneous, hierarchical, stepwise, and logistic. These are defined in separate entries in this dictionary.

Unfortunately there is little or no agreement regarding what sort of information should be reported in an article concerning the results of a regression analysis. Knapp (1994) has recently tried to remedy that situation.

The variables in a regression analysis are usually interval or ratio scales, but dichotomies can also be used if they have been generated by dummy coding or other ways of redefining nominal or ordinal variables.

Example: In nursing education research, interest might center on the predictability of grade point average in a master's degree program (Y) by some combination of undergraduate grade point average (X_1), the verbal score on the Graduate Record Examination (X_2), and the quantitative score on that exam (X_3). Polit and Hungler (1991, pp. 462-464) use this example in their discussion of multiple regression analysis, that is, regression analysis for which there is more than one independent variable. Two very popular multiple regression texts are Pedhazur (1982) and Cohen and Cohen (1983).

Reliability

Reliability is a technical term that has several meanings. As far as measurement is concerned, an instrument is called reliable if it produces *consistent* measures from time to time, from measurer to measurer, and so forth. But the term is also used in statistical analysis (a sample statistic is reliable if it doesn't vary much from sample to sample) and in engineering (a piece of equipment is reliable if it is unlikely to break down while it is being used). To make matters even more confusing, lay people use the term *reliability* in the same sense that the term *validity* (another very important measurement concept) is used by social scientists, for example, "The custodian is very reliable."

The reliability of a measuring instrument is usually determined by one or more of the following procedures:

1. Parallel forms (equivalence)—for tests that have two equivalent forms, say A and B, scores on Form A are compared with scores on Form B.
2. Test-retest (stability)—the same persons are measured on two separate occasions and the Time 1 scores are compared with the Time 2 scores.
3. Split halves (internal consistency)—the test is administered just once but for scoring purposes the scores on half of the test are correlated with the scores on the other half of the test (usually the odd-numbered questions vs. the even-numbered questions) and the Spearman-Brown formula is used to estimate the reliability of the entire test.
4. Coefficient alpha (internal consistency)—again the test is administered just once and a special formula is used to estimate reliability.

Researchers are often also interested in interrater reliability, referring to a variety of techniques for determining the reliability of the *scoring* of a test (it is actually the *objectivity* of measurement with which such techniques are concerned). Armstrong (1981) discusses one such technique.

There are competing theories regarding the reliability of measuring instruments, the most well known being the classical test theory of true scores and obtained scores (Carmines & Zeller, 1979; Nunnally & Bernstein, 1994). A true score on a variable is the measurement that a person *deserves* to get and would get if the instrumentation were perfectly reliable. An obtained score is the measurement that a person *does* get; it may or may not be equal to the corresponding true score. The difference between a person's obtained score and the corresponding true score is called an error score (or simply, an error). The errors are assumed to be *random* and not systematic.

It is essential to understand that the distinction between a true score and an obtained score is a matter of reliability and not validity (Knapp, 1985). Reliability deals with random errors, whereas validity deals with systematic errors. The measuring instrument may or may not be a valid device for operationalizing the construct of interest. That is a separate issue. A person's obtained score may be very close to his or her true score on a valid test or on an invalid test. It could also be very different from the true score for both kinds of tests.

Individual true scores are of course always unknown. But by making certain reasonable assumptions several interesting results can be demonstrated regarding groups of true scores. For example, the mean true score is equal to the mean obtained score and the correlation between true scores on one test and true scores on another test is equal to the correlation between the obtained scores divided by the square root of the product of the reliability coefficients (the so-called correction for attenuation).

Nursing researchers with a biophysiological bent tend to take a slightly different, yet still "quantitative," approach to reliability (see Engstrom, 1988; and DeKeyser & Pugh, 1990).

Example: If one were interested in determining the reliability of a test such as the Miller Analogies Test (a test often used for admission to graduate study), any or all of the above methods might be appropriate. The test does have several parallel forms; stability of scores from one time to the next might be of interest; it consists of 100 items for which split halves and/or coefficient alpha analysis might be desired; and although it is allegedly perfectly objective, because it can be machine scored, it might be interesting to see if two scorers using the same scoring key would have 100% agreement.

Qualitative researchers have tended to combine issues of reliability with those of validity. Validity is the concept that has received greater attention (Kirk & Miller, 1986). The idea of consistent measures as an expression of reliability is a part of research design, for example, testing and documenting reliability of fieldnotes or informants. Specific strategies to reduce threats to reliability are use of low-inference descriptors, verification of data through participants' review of findings or peer examination, and using a variety of data sources. The idea of stability, repeatability, or replicability as another type of reliability involves judging the clarity of written research reports. A study may be judged to be reliable if the reader can follow the "audit trail" (Lincoln & Guba, 1985) used in the research process and if another researcher (given similar data, perspective, and situation) could draw comparable conclusions. A research-generated theory may be judged to be reliable if it is applicable to similar situations over time.

Repeated-Measures Design

A repeated-measures design is a type of experimental design in which subjects are exposed to all of the treatments, in randomized order.

See **Experiment**.

Replication

The term *replication* has two different, though related, meanings in scientific research. Within an experimental study, especially those studies involving repeated-measures designs, each "subject" (person, rat, hospital, etc.) is called a replication, or replicate. But the more common usage is *across* studies, where a second study that is carried out on the same research problem is called a replication of the first study.

In that second sense of the term, replication studies have been both downplayed and encouraged. A doctoral student who would like to see if the results of X's study would be repeatable for a different sample of patients might be criticized for proposing an investigation that is "only" a replication of X's work. On the other hand, there is a constant cry for such studies because X's results might very well be unique to the particular situation that X chose to look at. (Perhaps the master's thesis is the ideal vehicle for replication studies?)

It is also not clear exactly what replication means in this second sense of the term. Must the second study duplicate every single aspect of the first study except one (e.g., the sample of subjects)? Or is it a replication study if it is merely an investigation of the same general research topic in a similar manner?

Example: A study of the effect of cigarette smoking on lung cancer in a highly industrialized environment would have to be replicated at least once in a pollution-free rural environment to get a better feel for whether the incidence of the cancer is linked with the cigarette smoking, with the pollution, or with some complicated confounding of the two.

147

Research

Research is a systematic process of investigation, the general purpose of which is to contribute to the body of knowledge that shapes and guides academic and/or practice disciplines. Research focused on the knowledge base, that is, the work of extending theory, may also be called *basic* or *fundamental research* in contrast to *applied research,* which is more concerned with using the knowledge generated by an investigation to develop practical approaches to problematic situations. In a practice discipline like nursing, the difference is often in emphasis rather than substance. To be of relevance to practice, research needs to accomplish both ends.

Research is sometimes compared with the *problem-solving* process. If applied research and basic or theory-linked research were placed at either end of a continuum, studies at the extreme "applied" end might be considered within the category of "problem solving." They would be concerned with concrete needs or problems in contrast with research problems that are theory driven and more general. Findings that result from problem solving pertain to the particular situation at hand, whereas the goal of research is to contribute to a discipline's knowledge base; that is to say, the use of research methods to investigate a problem does not necessarily produce scientific knowledge. However, there is increasing refinement in the application of research techniques across important types of studies such as quality assurance studies, evaluation research, need analysis, and policy research. The immediate utilitarian appeal of research procedures adapted for applied studies of this sort is that they provide investigators with powerful tools with which to address practical everyday concerns that arise in human service organizations and agencies.

Nursing is responsible for identifying the kinds of knowledge most valued as rationales for practice within and across care settings. Carper (1978) has described four important *patterns of knowing* as (a) empirical, (b) aesthetic, (c) personal, and (d) ethical. Emphasis in research has been on development of empirical knowledge, although Meleis (1991) asserts that nurse theorists have taken a more holistic approach that incorporates all ways of knowing in their views of nursing and nursing practice.

Empirics, "the science of nursing," specifies phenomena of interest in observable, measurable terms to describe, explain, and predict behavior and to validate or test theory. Empirical analytic studies fit within the perspective described in this dictionary as quantitative research. Qualitative research perspectives also are concerned with the empirical world. However, the approaches taken in qualitative research deal more with the meaning of subjective experience. There is more emphasis on aesthetics, "the *art* of nursing," that is expressive, empathetic, and concerned with individual perceptions and experiences; on personal knowledge (reflection, intuition, and understanding of use of self in interpersonal processes); and on ethical knowledge as a philosophical approach to reasoning about what ought to be.

In nursing theory and practice these four types of knowledge are interdependent. Different forms of investigation capture the ways in which they are distinct. For example, a phenomenological study (aesthetic/interpretation) or empirical hypothesis testing can be done without addressing the other forms of knowledge and how they are related. Empirical research methods have traditionally been recognized as the only legitimate (and the only "scientific") methods for generating knowledge. However, this view has been challenged by theorists and researchers who insist that methods for developing all areas of knowledge are essential to human science disciplines such as nursing and, therefore, must be equally legitimate. When methods for developing all patterns of knowing are equally recognized, the view of what constitutes "scientific research" is changed and expanded significantly. In this dictionary different research approaches are described along with some associated epistemological perspectives and concepts. It is not our intent to promote any one approach to research or theory development over others. Rather, we strongly believe that the advancement of nursing science and practice depends upon the successful integration of all patterns of knowing through a pluralistic approach to theorizing and research.

The plurality of views on what constitutes different research approaches also extends to notions about research as a systematic process. All research, whether of a quantitative or qualitative type, involves discipline and structure. However, the shape of the process varies according to the overall research perspective that guides the design of the project. Spradley (1980), in describing ethnographic research, made a helpful distinction between empirical-analytic studies' use of a *linear pattern* of investigation in contrast to the *cyclical pattern* followed in many qualitative studies. The linear pattern is the research sequence described in most standard research texts as "the" scientific approach (see, for example, Polit & Hungler, 1991). Research that follows a linear pattern proceeds in step-by-step fashion. (Sources differ in the actual number of steps, but it is the nature of the sequenc-

R

ing and the flow of the process that is being discussed here.) The process involves (a) defining a research problem, including reviewing related literature and developing a conceptual framework; (b) formulating a hypothesis (in some studies); (c) making operational definitions; (d) choosing or designing a research instrument and developing the study plan (research design, population, sampling method, and data management procedures); (e) drawing a sample and collecting data; (f) analyzing the data; (g) drawing conclusions; and (h) reporting the results, that is, the findings from the analysis, the conclusions, and the implications for practice and for future research. In research that follows this sequence the overall design (Steps a through d) is fixed prior to data collection; data analysis proceeds after data are collected; and analysis does not tend to lead to new questions and the collection of more data to be reported in that research project. Researchers determine what they are looking for in advance and do not deviate from preestablished procedures. Often pilot studies are conducted between Steps d and e to determine appropriateness of procedures and measuring instruments and to check for unanticipated problems. In some projects, maximum time and effort is expended on the research design, which, if well planned, facilitates a more rapid flow through the end phases of data collection and analysis.

Qualitative types of research that follow a cyclical process proceed in a spiral fashion through phases of simultaneous data collection and analysis that tend to refine and illuminate the originally stated research questions and thus guide future sampling and analysis procedures. (See, for example, the use of theoretical sampling in grounded theory research.) Statements of hypotheses and operational definitions are not characteristically a part of the research design. In theory-generating research, the placement of the findings and the conclusions of a study within the context of relevant literature may be a developing process throughout the project, with the theory statement and conceptual framework at the end rather than at the beginning of the research. The aspect of a phenomenon that remains to be discovered (culture, values, social process, essence—what an experience is like) cannot be precisely determined or known in advance. And the best procedures for drawing it out, likewise, may need to evolve as more about the phenomenon comes into view. In much qualitative research, understanding of the phenomenon comes in the final stages of the analysis and in the writing of final reports. Thus, maximal time and research effort shifts toward the later rather than the beginning phases of the research project with new insights often leading to new questions and collection of more data to complete the end account (see **Saturation**). Further, many qualitative researchers do not take any report of their research to be final, leaving it open to revision and further development. They may continue to work with the same data for years, drawing new and different analyses from them.

Nowhere in either the linear or the cyclical research process is there lack of concern for clear articulation of the research problem, placement of the problem with regard to relevant literature, attention to the conceptual or theoretical context, and methodological rigor of data collection and analysis techniques. Researchers following either pattern need to be able to design a research proposal that speaks to the above issues and that details with some precision the procedures and anticipated progress through each phase of the planned project. The contrast between linear and cyclical patterns is one of differences between modes of knowledge production where the content, emphasis, sequencing, degree of openness and flexibility, and rhythm of the work are varied to fit the epistemological assumptions and methods of the research tradition within which the researcher is functioning.

Increasingly, theory and research are viewed as interrelated activities rather than distinct entities. The relationship is often viewed as a spiral that revolves between theory-generating research of the qualitative type (primarily an inductive approach with the purpose of discovering and describing relationships inferred from an intensive study of human social situations) and theory-testing research of the quantitative type (primarily a deductive approach with the purpose of validating relational statements from theory, using an experimental or correlational design). Chinn and Kramer (1995) depict the interaction between theory and research as a spiral:

> If you begin with theory, research derived from the theory is used to clarify and extend the theory. If you begin with research, theory that is formed from the findings can be subsequently used to direct research. In order for this spiral process to continue, research must be conducted with the specific aim of contributing to theory development. (p. 143)

Munhall and Boyd (1993) describe a qualitative-quantitative cyclical continuum that also encourages increasing refinement of theories through expanding cycles of discovery-description-theory; hypothesis-validation-theory-*nuance*; and discovery-description-theory:

R

we would like to propose a nonlinear schema where qualitative descriptions would lead to a quantitative analysis (when that is appropriate), and, from that analysis, nuances for further qualitative study would be identified. For example, many studies statistically support the proposition that preoperative teaching reduces anxiety for the majority of preoperative patients. There are some patients, however, in whom such teaching increases anxiety. This is a nuance and calls us back to a qualitative study: "What about those patients?" We need now to discriminate further within our populations. Theories always need reevaluating, and the nuances or the exceptions often alert us to alternative or evolving ways of viewing phenomena. (pp. 59-60)

The above conceptualizations imply that theory refinement is dependent upon an interactive rather than a hierarchical relationship between different types of research. These authors present an enlarged overview of how the efforts of many researchers using diverse methods collectively and cooperatively build theory in a discipline. Their examples are not intended to illustrate typical or ideal research programs of individuals over time but, rather, research programs in the collective. Although they may have an equal appreciation for quantitative and qualitative modes of inquiry, many researchers favor one or the other in their own work and do not alternate between the two.

See **Evaluation Research, Need Analysis, Problem Solving, Qualitative Research, Quantitative Research,** and **Theory.**

Retention

In phenomenological research, retention involves bringing to remembrance and keeping in mind the details of a described experience.

See **Phenomenology.**

Retrospective Study

A retrospective study is a type of correlational research in which a search is made, after the fact, for one or more independent variables that are potential causes of the dependent variable(s). Such studies are also called causal-comparative studies or (by epidemiologists) case-control studies.

See **Case-Control Study** and **Correlational Research.**

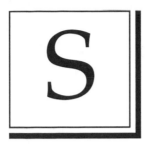

Sample

A sample is a subset of a population. It is often studied in preference to the entire population because of practical considerations such as cost and availability.

See **Inferential Statistics** and **Sampling**.

Sampling

Sampling is the process of selecting a subset of objects from a larger set (population) of objects.

Except for certain kinds of surveys, sampling tends to receive short shrift in nursing research. Yet from a scientific point of view it is hard to imagine anything more important than the representativeness of the sample upon which an investigation has been based.

Research samples can be probability samples or nonprobability samples, the former always being the more desirable. In probability sampling every object in the population of interest has a *known* probability of being drawn into the sample. A simple random sample is one for which the probability of selection of an object is *equal* to that for every other object. (The selection of a given object must also be independent of the selection of another object.)

But there are at least two other kinds of probability sampling. The first is stratified random sampling, whereby the population is divided into two or more subpopulations, or *strata*, and a simple random sample is selected from each *stratum*. In this way one can ensure that the sample is representative of the population with respect to at least one variable, namely the variable (sex, race, etc.) that produced the strata. For simple random sampling without stratification the sample is only *likely* to be representative. (A simple random sample of 25 people drawn from a large population that is 50% male and 50% female may, but probably will not, consist of all same-sex members.)

Another type of probability sampling is multistage cluster sampling. At the first stage, 10 large cities might be drawn at random; at the second stage, 2 hospitals might be drawn at random from each of the 10 cities; finally, all nurses at each of those 20 hospitals might be asked to participate in the research. This is quite different from having a "sampling frame" (list) of nurses and drawing a simple random sample of nurses from that sampling frame. The analysis of the data for the former case is also different (and more complicated) because between-hospital and between-city variation must be taken into account as well as between-nurse variation.

Nonprobability sampling includes all sampling procedures (quota sampling, volunteer sampling, "convenience" sampling, "snowball" sampling, "purposive" sampling) where chance plays no role in the determination of the actual constitution of the sample.

The following diagram may be helpful in distinguishing between probability and nonprobability sampling, and among their various subtypes:

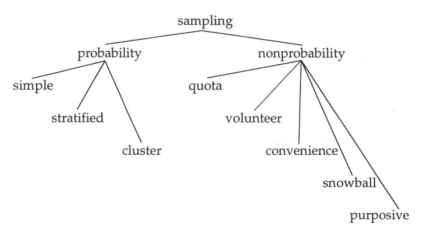

One type of sampling that could fall under either heading is systematic sampling, that is, sampling of "every *k*th" object. If the starting point in sampling from a list is chosen at random there is a probabilistic aspect. If not, that kind of sampling falls into the nonprobability category.

It is essential to distinguish among the terms *target population, sampled population, drawn sample,* and *responding sample.* The target population is the population that the researcher really cares about; it may or may not coincide with the population that is actually sampled. There may also be some attrition between the sample drawn and the responding sample. Some surveys regarding very sensitive topics such as attitudes toward abortion have extremely low response rates. The investigator may have drawn the sample at random from some accessible population, but it is the generalization from responding sample to target population that is of usual interest. Strictly speaking, statistical inference is only appropriate for generalizing from the drawn sample to the sampled population.

Finally, there is the matter of sample size. The extreme cases are easy. If you cannot afford to be wrong at all when generalizing from sample to population, you must take the whole population; if you don't mind being very wrong, take one object. But between $N = 1$ and $N =$ all, it depends on *how far wrong* you can afford to be, the assumed homogeneity of the population, the number of variables, and many other things. Fortunately there exist formulas and tables (e.g., Cohen, 1988) to help out.

Example: In a survey of nurses' smoking behavior, simple random sampling of the most recent ANA directory should provide a representative "snapshot" of such behavior by professional nurses (to the extent to which that directory mirrors the profession), particularly if the sample size is large (say 1000 or so), the response rate is good, and the questions are straightforward.

Sampling Distribution

A sampling distribution is a frequency distribution such as t, F, or chi-square that is used for making statistical inferences from samples to populations.

See **Inferential Statistics**.

Saturation

Saturation in qualitative research is a sense of closure that occurs when data collection ceases to provide new information and when patterns in the data become evident. Theoretical saturation is accompanied by personal saturation as the researcher concludes that the aims of the analysis have been carried out as far as possible.

See **Qualitative Research**.

Scale

As the term is most often used in social measurement, a scale is a group of items that "hang together." The term is also used in conjunction with the modifiers nominal, ordinal, interval, and ratio to provide one way of classifying variables. And there are bathroom scales for measuring weight, Fahrenheit and centigrade (Celsius) scales for measuring temperature, and so forth.

To determine the extent to which certain test items constitute a scale, a variety of techniques is available. The two most popular procedures are factor analysis and scalogram analysis. In the former procedure all of the inter-item correlations are obtained and subjected to a complicated statistical analysis that generates one or more "underlying" factors. Those items that have high "loadings" on the same factor go together to make up a scale (or perhaps a subscale). Scalogram analysis is similar, but the emphasis is on the coefficient of reproducibility, which is a measure of how well a group of items approximates what is called a Guttman scale (see separate entry).

A nominal scale is a variable such as religious affiliation for which measurement consists merely in designating a qualitative category (Catholic, Protestant, etc.) into which a person falls. An ordinal scale is a bit more precise and consists of a set of *ordered* categories (e.g., the traditional strongly agree, agree, undecided, disagree, and strongly disagree categories used in Likert scales). An interval scale, best exemplified by something like outdoor temperature in degrees centigrade (Celsius), is one step higher because the categories (−10, 0, +20, etc.) are not only ordered, but there is a meaningful unit (the degree) that is constant throughout the scale. A ratio scale is the highest level of measurement, and for such scales (e.g., physical force measured in dynes) there is a "real" zero point in addition to ordered categories with a constant unit. (The zero point for physical force is *no force*, whereas the zero point in degrees Celsius for outdoor temperatures is *not* no temperature; it is simply that rather arbitrary point at which water becomes ice.) The terms *nominal scale, ordinal scale, interval scale,* and *ratio scale* are due to Stevens (1946).

Polit and Hungler (1991) include several sections in their text that deal with scales in all of the above senses. Williamson et al. (1982)

provide a simple example of Guttman scaling and also a brief section on nominal, ordinal, interval, and ratio variables. Knapp authored two articles (1990, 1993) dealing with the often-subtle distinction between ordinal and interval scales and the controversy that such a distinction has engendered.

Example: A Toledo self-balancing *scale* yields weights that constitute data for a ratio *scale*.

Science

Although it is almost never defined in any textbook, science is best thought of as an activity that combines research (the advancement of knowledge) and theory (explanation for knowledge).

Some authors compartmentalize science in a variety of ways. One of the most common ways is basic science versus applied science. The term *basic science* refers to the study of phenomena from a purely epistemological standpoint, regardless of any practical applications the findings might happen to have. *Applied science,* as the term implies, is oriented toward the solution of practical problems. The distinction is easiest to see in mathematics (where some very important theorems have absolutely no real-world representations) and in biology (where studies involving animals are called basic and studies involving humans are called applied).

Although science = research + theory, not all scientists are both researchers and theorists. It is fairly common practice in many sciences for a relatively small number of scientists to do most or all of the theorizing and for the others to carry out research that either generates or tests such theories.

Example: Nursing is a science. Although some of its theories are "borrowed" from other disciplines, there *are* nursing theories, and there have been thousands of research investigations that have generated such theories and/or subjected them to empirical testing.

Secondary Analysis

Secondary analysis involves the creation of a research project based on a reanalysis of data previously collected for other purposes. There are a number of ways in which this research approach can be used effectively to produce new and important information. Research projects tend to yield more data than can be analyzed at one time. In addition to studying unanalyzed variables, the secondary investigator can test other aspects of relationships among variables or can examine particular subsamples. Different analytic techniques may be employed to reexamine the original design and research hypothesis if the researcher thinks that the original approach may have been inappropriate or weak. Data may also be organized differently for analysis; for example, the unit of analysis may be changed from distinct sets of individual responses to the aggregate, with individual responses merged and treated as a single unit, or vice versa. In addition, smaller or larger categories of data may be created that more closely relate to the current research interest or new hypothesis to be tested. The limitations of this approach involve those typically associated with use of existing data; that is, the secondary investigator has no control over how the data were collected, and in content, the data may not exactly suit the purposes of the proposed research.

Increasing use of computer technology has given rise to data banks that store survey data (although secondary analysis may also involve use of data collected by other means). Lists of data banks, which include both government and private sources, are obtainable (see, for example, McArt & McDougal, 1985). In the case of large-scale data sets, secondary analysis not only helps to extend the research potential of the original data but is also cost-effective:

> The policies regulating the public use of data vary from one organization to another, but it is not unusual for data to be provided to an interested researcher at about the costs for duplication plus handling. Thus, in some cases in which the gathering of the data involved an expenditure of thousands of dollars, reproduced materials may be supplied for less than 1% of the initial costs. (Polit & Hungler, 1991, p. 212)

In the case of smaller data sets, researchers sometimes indicate a willingness to make study data available to other investigators for the purpose of secondary analysis.

Kiecolt and Nathan (1985) have written an entire monograph devoted to the secondary analysis of survey data. A nursing research example of a secondary analysis is provided by Lucas et al. (1993).

Secondary Source

A secondary source is a source of data that consists of summarization of or commentary about primary data, such as writings or a life experience, by someone other than the person who produced the data or lived through the experience.

See **Primary Source**.

Semantic Differential

The semantic differential is a measurement strategy first introduced by Osgood, Suci, and Tannenbaum (1957) for assessing the connotative and denotative meanings of various concepts. The subject is given a number of concepts, such as love, ideal patient, and so forth, and asked to rate each concept on each of a number of bipolar scales, such as good/bad, strong/weak, and so forth. The purpose is to determine the distances between pairs of concepts in the "semantic space" formed by those scales. Those concepts that are close together in that space are things that are perceived as similar in meaning and those that are far apart are things that have very little in common with one another.

The study by Bowles (1986) is a good example of the use of the semantic differential in nursing research.

Semiotics

Semiotics (also called semiology) is the study of signs, or more generally, the study of patterned communication systems. It is associated with the theoretical perspective of structuralism, which holds that there are social structures (cultural symbols or myths) that are unobservable but generate observable social phenomena. These social structures do not exist in the real world and are not formed out of the subjective perceptions of informants. They are created by the analyst and are based on objective observations.

Structuralism, best described by the anthropologist Claude Levi-Strauss, represents an intellectual movement of French origin that includes scholars from the fields of anthropology, linguistics, literary criticism, and sociology. The point of structuralist analysis of cultural myths, symbols, or signs that make up written, verbal, or nonverbal forms of human communication is mainly to provide an understanding of conceptual activity; that is, the field falls within cognitive studies of the human mind.

From a semiotic point of view, everything in life has meaning and communicates something, for example, linguistic expressions, gestures, clothing and hair styles, greeting cards, film, photography, and forms of mass communication such as advertising or television. Cultural conventions determine how signs are organized into codes, which may be fairly obvious, such as particular fashions in dress, or may require detailed analysis to draw them out, such as cultural values. Semiotic interpretations represent a form of qualitative philosophical analysis that is deconstructive in nature. That is, it involves uncovering data layer by layer to expose the underlying premises and

159

covert communications that call overt messages and themes into question.

For further information on, and examples of, semiotic interpretation, see Barthes (1984), *Mythologies*, and (1986), *The Rustle of Language*; Derrida (1981), *Positions*; Hawkes (1977), *Structuralism and Semiotics*; Hebdige (1979), *Subculture: The Meaning of Style*; Manning (1987), *Semiotics and Fieldwork*; and Manning and Cullum-Swan (1994), *Narrative, Content, and Semiotic Analysis*.

Sensitivity

The term *sensitivity* has at least three different, though weakly related, meanings in nursing research. Polit and Hungler (1991) use the term in a *measurement* context. An instrument is said to be sensitive if it is capable of picking up fine distinctions in the measurement of a particular construct, for example, obesity. (A "test" of obesity that can only categorize people as "fat" or "skinny" is not very sensitive.)

In addition to this use of the term as a property of a measuring instrument, there are two *statistical* contexts in which the notion of sensitivity arises. The first of these is in hypothesis testing, where a procedure such as the analysis of covariance is called sensitive because if the null hypothesis is false, the use of that statistical technique gives the researcher a fairly high probability of arriving at the decision to reject it.

The second (and more common) statistical context in which the term *sensitivity* appears is in the analysis of the data for certain kinds of epidemiological research involving diagnostic testing. A distinction is made between the sensitivity of a diagnostic test (e.g., computerized tomography for detecting lung cancer) and the specificity of that test. Sensitivity is the fraction of a diseased group that the test successfully detects, and specificity is the fraction of a healthy group that the test successfully identifies as healthy. These definitions are equivalent to two terms used in statistical hypothesis-testing—the probability of *not* making a Type II error (often called the *power* of a test of statistical significance) and the probability of *not* making a Type I error. The terms *true positives* and *true negatives* are also equivalent, although the complementary terms *false positives* (Type I errors) and *false negatives* (Type II errors) are more frequently encountered in the literature.

Example (of this third meaning of the term *sensitivity*): A diagnostic test for AIDS that has a sensitivity of .99 is very good indeed for determining that a person who actually has AIDS is correctly identified as having the disease. Unfortunately, however, the higher the sensitivity the lower the specificity (all other things being equal), so such a test might also identify as having AIDS a fairly sizable fraction of people who do not have the disease.

Sequential Analysis

Sequential analysis is an approach to statistical inference in which a variable (rather than fixed) sample size provides the basis for inferences that are made as the data accumulate. In sequential hypothesis-testing three (rather than two) decisions are made at each stage of data analysis with respect to the null hypothesis under investigation: accept it, reject it, or keep sampling.

Sequential analysis is particularly appropriate for clinical nursing research where subjects are entered into the study one at a time, subjects are in short supply, and measurements are expensive. It has been shown that on average the sample size required to test a particular effect is smaller for sequential analysis than for traditional forms of statistical inference.

For a comprehensive article that describes sequential hypothesis-testing, see Brown, Porter, and Knapp (1993).

S

Simultaneous Regression

Simultaneous regression is a type of regression analysis in which all of the independent variables are "entered" into the analysis at the same time.

Zachariah (1994) used simultaneous regression analysis in a study of maternal-fetal attachment.

See **Regression Analysis**.

Snowball Sampling

Snowball sampling is a type of nonprobability sampling in which subjects initially selected recruit other subjects, who in turn recruit still other subjects, and so forth.

For an example of the use of snowball sampling in nursing research, see Hitchcock and Wilson (1992).

See **Sampling**.

Specificity

In epidemiological research *specificity* is a term used to define the fraction of subjects correctly identified by some diagnostic procedure to not have a particular disease.

See **Sensitivity**.

Split Halves

Split halves is a method for assessing the internal consistency reliability of a set of test items. The researcher administers the test only once but, for scoring purposes, splits the test into two halves (ideally randomly, but usually by odd-numbered and even-numbered test questions) and obtains a score for each subject on each half. The scores on one half are then correlated with the scores on the other half, and the Spearman-Brown formula is applied to that correlation, yielding an estimate of the test's reliability. This technique is closely associated with Cronbach's coefficient alpha (which is the average of all possible split-half reliabilities) but is used less often in nursing research than alpha.

See **Reliability**.

Spurious Relationship

A spurious relationship is a relationship between two variables that vanishes when a third variable is taken into account.

Example: There is a very high positive correlation between height and reading ability of elementary school children. However, when age is taken into account (e.g., by the technique of partial correlation) that relationship is reduced very close to zero, because it is age that is "driving" both variables.

Stakeholders

In some types of investigation, people recruited into the study are not considered to be "subjects." Rather, because they are seen as partners in the research process, they are called respondents, participants, or stakeholders. The term *stakeholder* is common to emancipatory forms of inquiry, such as feminist research. Here it implies an open, nonexploitive researcher-participant relationship characterized by equality and mutuality. *Stakeholders* also is used to refer to participants in evaluation studies, where groups and individuals may be recognized as having vested interests in the program under review.

Standard Deviation

The standard deviation of a set of data for a variable is a descriptive statistic that summarizes the amount of variability around the mean. It is calculated by finding the mean of the squared deviations (differences) from the mean and then taking the square root. (The quantity obtained before taking the square root is called the variance; the standard deviation is the square root of the variance.) It can take on

S

values from 0 (no variability at all) to one half of the range (maximum variability). It should always be reported whenever the mean is reported, because two frequency distributions could have the same mean but quite different standard deviations and therefore indicate different amounts of variability with respect to that mean.

Some authors of statistics textbooks define the standard deviation in a slightly different way; they divide by one less than the number of "scores," rather than the actual number of "scores," before extracting the square root. The reasons for this are very complicated (see, for example, Munro & Page, 1993, p. 25).

See **Range** and **Variance**.

Statistic

A statistic is a descriptive index for a sample, such as a sample mean, a sample standard deviation, or a sample correlation coefficient. It is contrasted with a parameter, which is the corresponding descriptive index for the entire population.

See **Parameter** and **Sample**.

Stepwise Regression

Stepwise regression is a type of regression analysis that is different from, but often confused with, hierarchical regression.

In stepwise regression the independent variables are "entered" sequentially not according to any theory but strictly on the basis of statistical significance.

Narsavage and Weaver (1994) used stepwise regression analysis in their study of predictors of chronic obstructive pulmonary disease.

See **Regression Analysis**.

Stratified Random Sampling

Stratified random sampling is a type of random sampling in which the population is divided into subpopulations or "strata" on the basis of one or more variables and a simple random sample is drawn from each "stratum."

See **Sampling**.

Structural Equation Modeling

Structural equation modeling is an extension of path analysis to the situation in which both measured variables (sometimes called "manifest" variables) and unmeasured variables (the underlying "latent" variables, or factors) are of interest. The model has two parts: (a) the measurement model, in which the relationships between the manifest variables and their underlying latent counterparts are assessed; and (b) the structural model, in which the relationships between the latent variables are of prime concern.

The computer packages LISREL and/or EQS are usually employed to study both parts of the model. Pedhazur (1982) and the articles by Boyd, Frey, and Aaronson (1988), and by Aaronson, Frey, and Boyd (1988) are good references for understanding the basic concepts of structural equation modeling.

The studies by Johnson et al. (1993) and by Lusk et al. (1994) both used structural equation modeling, the former with LISREL and the latter with EQS.

Subject

In social research *subject* has a very special meaning, to wit, the person who is being studied. (If there is more than one person, they are called, naturally enough, subjects.) The abbreviations S (for subject) and Ss (for subjects) are very commonly used, particularly in the psychological literature, along with E and Es for experimenter(s).

Infrahuman animals used in basic research are occasionally also called subjects, but if inanimate things (hospital, county, etc.) are the units of analysis some other term is usually employed. A term sometimes used interchangeably with subject is *object*, which is indeed strange as the two words have quite different meanings in English grammar (subject-predicate-object) and in common parlance (e.g., a school subject such as history or the object of someone's affection).

Some people find the term *subject* a bit demeaning (conveying the impression that the person[s] being studied should be regarded as subservient to the researcher) and suggest the less pejorative term *participant*. Participants who in some types of research are viewed as partners and co-investigators are sometimes referred to as stakeholders.

Most universities in which scientific research is carried out now have "human subjects" committees whose responsibility is to oversee the protection of the rights of study participants through informed consent, anonymity, freedom to withdraw from the study without retaliation, and so forth. Although the paperwork involved is often enormous, the ethical considerations are given the priority they justly deserve.

Survey

The term *survey* has two equally common meanings. Half of the scientific community defines a survey as research that involves questionnaires and/or interviews and large numbers of respondents. The other half of the scientific community defines a survey as any research based on a probability sample, that is, a sample drawn from a population in such a way that every object has a known probability of being selected.

For those who adopt the latter definition, the survey may or may not involve questionnaires or interviews, and may or may not involve large numbers of participants. For example, a study in which a simple random sample of 112 adult males are weighed would be regarded by this "camp" as survey research, whereas the questionnaire/interview "camp" would call that sort of study something else ("descriptive research" is a popular catch-all category).

Surveys that involve a series of questions in interview or questionnaire format are usually conducted for the general purpose of obtaining information about practices, opinions, attitudes, and other characteristics of people. Survey researchers typically collect a broad range of demographic data on participants' backgrounds as well. Although these data may not be central to the study, they may help to explain the study findings, because background characteristics frequently can be linked with behavioral and attitudinal patterns. The most basic function of a survey is description, although explanation of why people behave or believe as they do and prediction of responses with regard to the variable(s) of interest may be additional objectives.

A number of designs may be used in surveys. The main concerns are with sampling procedures, sample size, and instrument validity and reliability. Researchers try to obtain as large a sample as necessary to minimize sampling error and to allow for a certain percentage of nonresponse. Careful construction of interview schedules and questionnaires, and pilot testing of these instruments, is essential. A pilot study based on a small preliminary sample can alert the researcher to questions that may need to be changed or deleted, additional questions that should be included, or other logistical revisions.

An advantage of surveys is that large amounts of data can be amassed. A disadvantage is that the actual information content can be fairly superficial. The researcher must determine if study interests are best served by an extensive survey focused on selected variables or by an intensive examination (case study) of more variables with a small sample or single subject. Because the investigator usually has little control over the research situation, causal relationships are more difficult to establish in surveys than in true experiments. However, carefully designed surveys are almost always objective, are a good source for hypotheses, and can suggest directions for further research.

Example (of a study that would satisfy both definitions): A researcher interested in the smoking behavior of nurses might draw a probability sample of 1,000 nurses from the population of nurses listed in the latest edition of the ANA directory and send out a questionnaire to each of those nurses asking for information regarding whether or not they smoke cigarettes, how many they smoke, and so forth.

Symbolic Interaction

Symbolic interaction is a theoretical perspective associated with the "Chicago school," that is, the University of Chicago Department of Sociology and scholarly work emanating from it for over 20 years between World War I and the mid-1930s. During this period the Chicago school dominated American sociology. Symbolic interaction was one of many emphases in Chicago sociology at this time. It originated with the social psychology of George Herbert Mead. From 1894 until his death in 1931, Mead taught courses in the philosophy department at Chicago that were attended by many graduate students in sociology. His ideas so profoundly affected them that they put together their lecture notes and published a posthumous volume under his name. Symbolic interaction was created from this effort and from other input from faculty in the Department of Sociology. Herbert Blumer actually coined the phrase and advocated symbolic interaction in the Meadian tradition at Chicago in the 1940s and 1950s.

Symbolic interaction was an alternative to the dominance of functionalism and social systems theory with their emphasis on equilibrium models. These latter perspectives focused on explaining social behavior according to the role or function it served in the larger society but neglected to account for individual motives and the meanings people give to their actions.

In Mead's philosophy, a person's sense of self emerges through social interaction. The relationship between self and society is an ongoing process of symbolic communication. A sense of self develops as people (a) imagine themselves in other social roles (seeing themselves as through the eyes of others and internalizing the attitudes of the generalized other), (b) anticipate the responses of others, and (c) act in accordance with the meaning that things (other people, ideas, events, objects, or situations) have for them. Thus, through thought and action, people are continuously creating social reality. But they are rarely aware of this process that goes along with the flow of everyday life.

Symbolic interactionists advocated methods that would allow researchers to explore the meanings hidden in the social world of the individual. Grounded theory method, developed by Glaser and Strauss (1967), takes a symbolic interactionist perspective. The Chicago school ethnographic studies of urban life also were linked with this perspective in their concern with identity formation, which was thought to be the result of people's self-perceptions in combination with how they thought others viewed them. Erving Goffman (1922-1982), a student of Blumer at Chicago, developed dramaturgical analysis as a variation of symbolic interaction. Interpretation of social behavior takes a view of life as theater. The assumption is that when people interact, they want to manage others' impressions of themselves. Consequently, they give performances, enact parts or routines, make use of environment for setting and props, and control what is stage front and backstage (hidden from the audience). The central concern in Goffman's work is the self in society. The drama of everyday life lies in its fragility and its potential for disruption by misunderstandings, embarrassments, uncertainties, and similar tensions that routinely occur in face-to-face encounters of varying duration. Systems and people in systems are constantly working to maintain mechanisms that prevent tensions from becoming too severe and overwhelming the balance needed to sustain social interaction.

The symbolic focus on role and communication has influenced studies of (a) the sociology of illness behavior, (b) patient-care provider interaction, and (c) the role of social factors in health care systems.

For additional information see Blumer (1969); Ditton (1980); Goffman (1959, 1961, 1963, 1967, 1971); Mead (1934, 1938, 1959); Meltzer, Petras, and Reynolds (1975); and Rose (1962).

See **Grounded Theory.**

Systematic Sampling

Systematic sampling is a type of sampling in which every *k*th (where *k* is some convenient number) member of the population is selected into the sample.

Floyd (1993) has written a very comprehensive article on systematic sampling.

See **Sampling.**

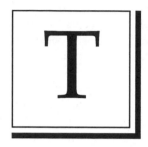

t Test

The *t* test is a very popular test of statistical significance for assessing the difference between two sample means. The samples are usually independent, but occasionally they are dependent (correlated, matched, paired).

Janke (1994) used a *t* test (one tailed) in one of the analyses she carried out regarding the development of an instrument for predicting breast-feeding attrition.

See **Test of Significance**.

Taxonomy

A taxonomy is a classification scheme for defining or gathering together various phenomena. Taxonomies range in complexity from simple dichotomies such as types of nursing research (e.g., experiments and nonexperiments) to hierarchical structures such as those for the objectives in the cognitive, affective, and psychomotor domains of nursing education cited by Waltz, Strickland, and Lenz (1991). These authors use the term in a very restrictive sense to suggest that the creation of a taxonomy will provide a standard lexicon for communication about the phenomena of interest. See, for example, Kolcaba's (1991) taxonomy of the concept "comfort."

Other authors use the term heuristically. In these instances creation of taxonomies facilitates the organization and presentation of research findings. However, there is no intent to move toward a standard terminology. See, for example, Hogan and DeSantis's (1992) taxonomy of the adolescent sibling bereavement process and Powers's (1988a, 1988b, 1991, 1992) taxonomy of types of nursing-home residents.

Test of Significance

A test of significance is a statistical hypothesis-testing procedure for determining the extent to which a particular sample result may be attributable to chance.

Such a test involves the postulation of a null (chance) hypothesis (e.g., that there is no relationship between X and Y) and an alternative hypothesis (usually arising from some sort of theory) regarding the population of interest. A sample is drawn from the population, a statistic is calculated for that sample, and a decision is made to reject or not to reject the null hypothesis. If the null hypothesis is rejected, the sample result is said to be statistically significant.

If a true null hypothesis is rejected (the researcher never knows whether it is true or false, but must entertain both possibilities), a Type I error is said to have been made. If a false null hypothesis is not rejected, a Type II error is said to have been made. The probabilities of making these kinds of errors are called alpha errors (Type I) and beta errors (Type II) because of the Greek symbols used to denote them. The probability of making a Type I error is also called the level of significance. The complement of the probability of making a Type II error, that is, 1 – beta, is called the power of the test of significance.

The researcher usually tries to keep both alpha and beta small (conventionally around .05 or so), but unfortunately as one decreases the other increases, all other things being equal. The only way to minimize both of them is to draw a very large sample size (take a bigger "chunk" out of the population). That can be expensive and often leads to statistically significant but not very important results.

If the alternative hypothesis is "directional" or "one sided" (e.g., there is an inverse relationship between X and Y), a "one-tailed test" is called for. If the alternative hypothesis is nondirectional (e.g., there is a relationship between X and Y), a "two-tailed test" is called for. Those names derive from the area of the sampling distribution in which the "rejection region" (alpha region) for the test is located.

T

The most commonly encountered tests of significance are the *t* test for the difference between two sample means, the analysis of variance *F* test for several sample means, the analysis of covariance *F* test for "adjusted" sample means, and the chi-square test of the relationship between two nominal variables.

All four of those procedures involve the concept of "degrees of freedom" (df), a term associated with the corresponding sampling distributions (*t*, *F*, or chi-square) that are used to carry out the tests.

Example: If the null hypothesis of no relationship between age and pulse rate were tested against the alternative hypothesis of an inverse relationship between the two, and a sample of 1000 observations yielded a correlation coefficient of −.08, the null hypothesis would be rejected in favor of the alternative, and the result would be statistically significant at the .01 level, but the finding would undoubtedly not be regarded as very important because the sample correlation is so close to zero.

Test-Retest

Test-retest is a procedure for assessing the reliability (stability) of a measuring instrument.

See **Reliability**.

T

Theorem

A theorem is a conclusion that is drawn from axioms as premises in a formal logical deductive reasoning format. Theorems and axioms pertain to the science of mathematics and are considered to be less tentative than other types of propositional statements.

See **Theory**.

Theoretical Sampling

Theoretical sampling is a data-gathering approach used in grounded theory and consistent with other qualitative methods. As data are concurrently collected and analyzed, the researcher decides what further data and data sources are needed to develop the emerging theory.

See **Grounded Theory**.

Theory

A theory is a set of statements that tentatively describe, explain, or predict relationships between concepts that have been systematically selected and organized as an abstract representation of some phenomenon. Concepts, sometimes called the "building blocks of theory," are the major ideas expressed by the theory and may be described as being located on a continuum from empirical to abstract (Kaplan, 1964; Chinn & Kramer, 1995). Concept analysis and testing of theoretical relationships through research involve defining concepts in relation to their empirical indicators or referents (those properties of concepts that can be verified). The means to accomplish this may be fairly direct in the case of concrete concepts (e.g., sex, weight, height), but abstract concepts will involve more indirect measures and multiple empirical indicators.

> Self-esteem is an example of a highly abstract concept for which there are no direct measures. The instruments or tools that are developed to assess self-esteem depend on theoretic definitions serving a specific purpose and are built on multiple behavioral responses that experts agree are associated with that concept. . . . Each behavioral trait contained in the tool can be considered as partial indicators of self-esteem. When the composite behaviors are built into an assessment tool, it is usually a more adequate indicator for the abstract concept than any one behavior taken alone. The composite score obtained from the tool is then considered to be a measurement constructed as an empiric indicator. (Chinn & Kramer, 1995, pp. 59-60)

Propositions are statements about the relationships between two or more concepts. Some specific types of propositions are postulates, premises, and axioms, which in a formal logical deductive format are introductory propositional statements. Axioms as premises are presumed to be true, in contrast to the tentative nature of most propositions. Other types of propositions are theorems, hypotheses, and laws, which in a chain of logical deductive reasoning are concluding propositional statements. Theorems are derived from axioms and more usually pertain to the science of mathematics. Because axioms as premises connote a greater degree of certainty, theorems also will be considered as less tentative than hypotheses (Floyd, 1983). Hypotheses are propositional statements that are tested by means of systematic research approaches. Supported hypotheses may also serve as premises in deductive arguments, where they lend a higher degree of soundness to conclusions than do untested premises. Propositions in theories are sometimes referred to as "lawlike" or as "laws of interaction." This is with reference to the logical development of theories, where it is expected that propositions will follow a clearly identifiable

171

line of reasoning from initial premises to conclusion. It is not intended to imply that all propositions are "laws" in the scientific sense. Patterns of relationships that have become widely accepted by virtue of repeated validation through research may be called laws. A law is a propositional statement that is highly generalizable, that is, consistently supported and therefore not tentative (Chinn & Kramer, 1995, p. 216). In comparison to the physical sciences, the social/human sciences have relatively few laws.

The tentative nature of theory is an important notion to appreciate, particularly as it relates to the foregoing discussion of the definitional linkages of theoretical concepts with empirical reality and the sequencing, testing, and credibility of propositional statements. Theory is not reality; it is an abstraction of reality based on assumptions about the true nature of the phenomenon in question that cannot be proven or disproven. The degree of support that may be found for a theory relies on applying various forms of reasoning to test the logic of propositional statements and validating associated hypotheses through research.

Theory creation in any discipline is a "living thing" with philosophical roots and historical traditions that produce various schools of thought. These schools of thought at times complement and at other times compete with one another. To some degree, then, every "conceptual" or "theoretical" position taken in a discipline will have historical antecedents. Identifying historical roots can do much to explain assumptions on which current thinking rests and leads to judgments regarding whether or not those assumptions are still valid. Most disciplines do not pay sufficient attention to this aspect of their "theory base." Thinkers and writers from Nightingale to the present have created a rich heritage for nursing by articulating concerns of the discipline and suggesting ways in which the profession might define its own domain. Central personalities have been identified in recent times as "nurse theorists." The majority of early nurse theorists had no intention of constructing a theory per se. Their writing combines philosophical treatises on the nature of nursing with heuristic devices to help nurses develop an organized approach to client assessment and care planning. Some, in this latter capacity, have served as bases for curricula in nursing education. Roy, King, and Newman have made conscious efforts to derive theories from their earlier work. Others, such as Rogers, support extension and testing of their thinking through the research efforts of colleagues.

Theory building is a complex, time-consuming process that can cover a number of developmental stages or phases from inception of the main concepts, either through research or through logical processes, to testing of theoretical propositions (hypothesis testing) through research. There has been disagreement over *when* in this process of theory building a particular thesis on, or conceptualization of, some phenomenon may be called a theory. Some authors, for example, Meleis (1991), have advocated an interpretation of the term that would allow for analysis of theoretical thinking at any point in the process of theory building. Others have argued that a systematic and clear linkage of conceptualization with procedures of scientific research has to be demonstrated for there to be a theory—that is, a theory has to be testable (Roy & Roberts, 1981; Newman, 1979).

Theory can be classified according to its purpose or the type of knowledge generated. Some writers think that in the practice sciences, the purposes of theory should go beyond the description, explanation, and prediction associated with scientific theory. The terms *prescriptive theory* and *practice theory* are sometimes used interchangeably to indicate a higher level of theorizing: " To understand, explain, predict, and prescribe nursing phenomena and nursing care, nurses should develop practice theories that emanate from the discipline and guide the discipline's actions . . . the ultimate goal is to develop theories to change situations. Therefore, theories that stress change as their goal are practice theories" (Meleis, 1991, p. 171).

Some theory designations refer to scope/breadth or the range of phenomena with which the theory deals. Theory may be classified as narrow range (atomistic, micro, molecular), middle/midrange, or broad range (macro, holistic, grand). Criteria for evaluating the scope of a theory vary across disciplines, and within disciplines there may be little consensus on how to apply these classifications or on what type is most desirable. Arguments have been put forth in nursing for grand theories that attempt to account for the total range of nursing activities in order to define boundaries for nursing science and identify common concerns of nurses functioning in different practice settings. Opposing arguments call for narrow- or middle-range theories dealing with more limited aspects of nursing associated with nursing specialty areas, such as rehabilitation nursing, or with particular care problems, such as pain. Another viewpoint is that the diverse interests and concerns of nursing require theories of varying scope and complexity.

Metatheory is an additional type of theory that does not generate any of the kinds of theory discussed above. Rather, metatheory is theory about theory and is concerned with generating knowledge and debate within a discipline around broad issues, such as the nature of theory in general, the types of theory needed by the discipline, and the most suitable criteria for evaluating theories. The metatheoretical literature is extensive and includes many viewpoints on nursing as a science and nursing as a practice discipline as well as opinions on the best approaches to theory construction and evaluation.

Theory may be further defined according to the process by which it is derived. A theory statement may evolve *as a result of* research (theory-generating research) that typically employs an inductive approach focused on discovery and description of experience and observed real-world events. Already constructed theory may be tested *through* research (theory-testing research) that typically employs a deductive approach focused on measurement of the constructs contained in the theory. (See the discussion of the relationship between theory and research in Chinn & Kramer, 1995, Chapter 8.)

Armchair theory is a type of theory derived not from research but from thought processes that employ either rules of logic or reasoned argument. On one hand, the term is often used pejoratively to imply that armchair theorists have a casual speculative approach to their subject matter and evidence a lack of concern for scientific method. Both Chinn and Kramer (1995) and Dubin (1978), on the other hand, defend "armchair" activities (the cognitive processes involved in concept analysis and construction of theoretical relationships) as being a legitimate and necessary part of scientific inquiry: "It is meaningless for empirical researchers to accuse theorists of being armchair philosophers. . . . Just because a theorist does not himself make the empirical tests of his models does not permit him to be condemned on the assumption that he does not want such tests made" (Dubin, 1978, p. 217).

Finally, theory may be defined in relationship to the discipline in which it originates and may be further associated with the name of its originator. Thus nursing theory is distinguished from psychological theory, educational theory, or anthropological theory; and references are made to Roy's theory or Freud's theory. This practice of labeling theories has affected nursing in two ways. First, there has been a tendency to view the association of someone's name with a theory as a sign of personal ownership. Therefore, there has been

T

reluctance on the part of nurses to criticize, test, and modify what is seen to be the "property" of another.

Second, there has arisen a distinction between "borrowed theory," defined as knowledge developed by other disciplines but used by nurses, and "unique theory," defined as knowledge developed from the unique perspective of nursing. Donaldson and Crowley (1978) argue that it is impossible to "borrow" knowledge from other disciplines because each has its own "unique" perspective, and therefore discussion of borrowed versus unique theory raises false issues.

Stevens (1984) coined the term *shared theory*: "Borrowed theories remain borrowed as long as they are not adapted to the nursing milieu and the nursing image of man. Once such theories have been adapted to the nursing milieu, it is logical to refer to these boundary overlaps as shared knowledge rather than as borrowed theories" (p 95). The idea of shared knowledge is probably closer to the reality of scientific life. Although the notion of "borrowing" knowledge persists in nursing, there appears to be increasing acceptance of the idea that scientific knowledge belongs to the scientific community and to society at large and is not the property of individuals or disciplines:

> Knowledge once generated by a discipline becomes the property of the public and may be used for whatever purposes it serves and by any academic discipline. Second, and more important, when theory or individual concepts from another discipline are used in nursing, the theory may become altered and advanced (Hardy, 1978). Concepts from the general pool of knowledge, regardless of source, may be found to be useful in nursing because they describe and explain human behavior relevant to the restoration and maintenance of health. (Christman & Johnson, 1981, p. 18)

> There are no divisions of knowledge in the real world. It is we who delineate certain areas of information as "belonging" to certain fields. The possessors of knowledge are those people who understand it and are aware of how to make use of it in appropriate and creative ways. (Downs, 1979, p. 72)

See also Stevens Barnum (1994) for further discussion of boundary issues in theory development associated with differentiation of nursing from other disciplines as well as for excellent coverage of analysis, application, and evaluation of nursing theory.

T

Thick Description

The concept of thick description, originated by Geertz (1973), is often used as a criterion for good ethnographic writing. It refers to the nature of the informational base that is needed for interpretation and understanding of culture and experience:

> A thin description simply reports facts, independent of intentions or circumstances. A thick description, in contrast, gives the context of the experience, states the intentions and meanings that organized the experience, and reveals the experience as a process. . . . The intent is to create the conditions that will allow the reader, through the writer, to converse with (and observe) those who have been studied. (Denzin, 1994, p. 505)

The analytic and interpretive qualities of thickly described experiences contribute depth to ethnographic writing and help to establish the credibility of the research.

See **Ethnography**.

Triangulation

Triangulation is a term used in a number of fields, such as surveying, radio broadcasting, astronomy, and navigation, to describe

> the process of determining the distance between points on the earth's surface, or the relative position of points, by dividing up a large area into a series of connected triangles, measuring a base line between two points, and then locating a third point by computing both the size of the angles made by lines from this point to each end of the base line and the length of these lines. (*Webster's New World Dictionary, Second College Edition*, 1974)

Other terms that have been used to describe triangulation as a practice or approach in research include multiple operationalism; convergent operationalism; operational delineation; convergent validation (in educational and psychological testing—see Campbell & Fiske, 1959); and corroboration, cross-validation, and multiple validation procedures (in qualitative research—see Becker, 1958).

Triangulation of data is used in qualitative studies as a way of confirming new information as it occurs over the course of data collection (Lincoln & Guba, 1985). This might involve seeking multiple and different information sources or using different data-collection techniques to obtain the information (interview, observation, questionnaire, testing). Confirmation by use of different investigators occurs when a team approach to field study is being used and when it includes regular opportunities for team members to interact, share, question, and reflect upon one another's observations and insights based on the unfolding body of evidence:

> The use of different investigators, a concept perfectly feasible for the conventionalist, runs into some problems in the naturalistic context. If the design is emergent, and its form depends ultimately on the particular interaction that the investigator has with the phenomena . . . then one could not expect corroboration of one investigator by another. The problem is identical to that of expecting replicability for the sake of establishing reliability. However, the naturalist sees it as perfectly possible to use multiple investigators as part of a team, with provisions being made for sufficient intrateam communication to keep all members moving together. (Lincoln & Guba, 1985, p. 307)

A number of qualitative researchers routinely validate information by various means but do not use, or prefer not to use, the term *triangulation*. Some researchers think that triangulation in the multiple operational sense ("the convergence function") is especially relevant in development of instruments and measurement of discrete constructs. Other researchers use the term triangulation to refer to a multistrategy approach to achieve completeness (Breitmayer, Ayres, & Knafl, 1993). Contextual validation that involves a multistrategy or multitheory approach is a design issue that does not carry the same sense of triangulation as a means of cross-validation. Concern has been expressed about the need for accuracy and consistency when using a multiple-method approach; for example, one should not combine methods that rest on different assumptions (Leininger, 1994). See also Morse's (1991a) article for articulation of principles underlying the use of methodological triangulation when combining qualitative and quantitative methods.

There is no clear agreement on the meaning and purposes of triangulation in research. It is used in very different ways. Therefore, researchers who use this approach must specify its meaning and purpose in relation to their work and cite the literature that is consistent with that orientation.

For a particularly good summary of triangulation see Kimchi, Polivka, and Stevenson (1991). See also Reed (1991), P. E. Stevens (1994), and Wilson and Hutchinson (1991).

True Experiment

A true experiment is an experiment that is characterized by manipulation, random assignment, and other controls.

See **Experiment**.

True Score

A true score is a score that a subject "deserves" to get on a test. It may differ from the score she or he actually obtains, however, due to the unreliability of the measuring instrument.

See **Reliability**.

Two-Tailed Test

A two-tailed test is a test of statistical significance in which a null hypothesis is pitted against a nondirectional alternative hypothesis.

See **Alternative Hypothesis**, **Null Hypothesis**, and **Test of Significance**.

Type I Error

In a test of statistical significance a Type I error is defined as the rejection of a true null hypothesis.

See **Test of Significance**.

Type II Error

In a test of statistical significance a Type II error is defined as the nonrejection ("acceptance") of a false null hypothesis.

See **Test of Significance**.

T

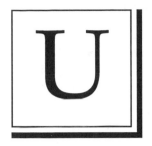

Unit of Analysis

The term *unit of analysis* has at least two different meanings in research. The first and more common meaning is the "thing" for which measurements have been obtained and subsequently subjected to data analysis. The unit might be a person (a patient or a nurse, for example), a hospital, a city, or virtually anything.

Occasionally the data may only be available for one unit of analysis, such as the hospital, but the researcher's interest may be in some other unit, such as the patient. Suppose that the research question is: "What is the relationship between amount of Demerol used and amount of reduction in pain?" For each of a number of *hospitals* we might know how much Demerol is dispensed each day and what percentage of the patients who take it each day actually experience pain reduction. But that is probably the wrong unit. We would like to know for each *patient* how much Demerol was used and whether or not she or he experienced any reduction in pain. If the *hospital* measurements are analyzed and the interpretation is made for a *patient*, a serious error could be committed, because the relationship could be quite different if the data were analyzed for individual patients. (Such an error is called an "ecological fallacy.")

Some authors (e.g., Polit & Hungler, 1991) use the term *unit of analysis* in a different sense. In content analysis the term is applied to the type of quantity being measured rather than the type of object on which the measurement is based.

Example: "What is the relationship between the heights and the weights of twins?" is a very difficult research question to answer because the unit of analysis could be an individual person or a pair of persons (if the latter, whose height and whose weight would be used?) and the two approaches could produce quite different results.

Unobtrusive Research

Unobtrusive research is research that is carried out on people who are unaware that they are being studied. It can take a variety of forms ranging from research involving hidden hardware (e.g., bedroom "bugging" for the purpose of studying sexual behavior) to archival research involving public records (e.g., birth certificates for studying the relationship between mother's age and baby's birth weight).

There is an entire book devoted to unobtrusive research (Webb, Campbell, Schwartz, Sechrest, & Grove, 1981). The principal advantages of such research are the lack of artificiality in what is studied and the inability of the subjects to refuse to cooperate in the research. The principal disadvantages are ethical ones (there are some serious moral and legal problems associated with bedroom bugging, for example), but for certain unobtrusive procedures there also are some sticky methodological problems. In a study of fascination with baby nurseries carried out by measuring smudges on the glass, you never know whether the smudges have been made by the same person spending a great deal of time watching the babies or by several persons all spending a short amount of time each. The same holds true if you want to use the amount of wear and tear on library books as a measure of their popularity. (There is also the additional problem, of course, that a particular book may be badly worn but never actually read!)

Some observational research is unobtrusive, but much is not. It is more common for anthropologists, sociologists, and so forth to obtain the explicit permission of the "observees" than it is for them to carry out their observations without the knowledge of the subjects being studied. The researchers are often participant observers and as such they usually cannot make their observations unobtrusively. (See Williamson et al., 1982, p. 212, for a well-known counterexample, *Tally's Corner*).

As far as the advancement of knowledge regarding a particular phenomenon is concerned, a fruitful strategy might be to combine both obtrusive (e.g., interview) and unobtrusive (e.g., archival) approaches in order to get a double "fix" on the problem. This strategy is sometimes called *triangulation*.

Example: For many years people who took standardized multiple-choice tests were asked to blacken in the space between vertical dotted lines when recording their answers. More recently they have been asked to blacken in small ovals. Does it matter? A very nice unobtrusive (and perfectly ethical) controlled experiment could be carried out by randomly distributing answer sheets to a group of people being tested, with half of them getting the vertical dotted lines and the other half getting the ovals. Neither subgroup would know that everyone was not getting the same response form, much less that they were participating in an experiment, thereby avoiding the dreaded Hawthorne Effect (see separate entry) that can often plague obtrusive research.

U

V

Validity

Validity is one of the two most important characteristics of a measuring instrument (the other is reliability). An instrument is said to be a *valid* way of operationalizing a construct if it really does measure that construct.

The literature is replete with procedures for determining whether or not, or to what extent, an instrument is valid, but they are all subsumed under three general types:

1. *Content validity* is concerned with the subjective determination of validity, usually by some sort of expert judgment, but alternatively or additionally by the persons being measured (the term face validity is used in the latter case).

2. In *criterion-related validity*, the measures obtained are compared with some external criterion that has itself already been judged to be valid (the "gold standard"). Some authors use the terms *concurrent validity* and *predictive validity* to distinguish between situations where the criterion data are gathered at about the same time as the measures for the instrument whose validity is in question and situations where the criterion data are gathered later.

3. *Construct validity* is concerned with theoretically based relationships that should pertain between measures produced by the instrument and measures of the same and other constructs.

Campbell and Fiske (1959) used the terms *convergent validity* and *discriminant validity* to refer to relationships with alleged measures of the same construct and relationships with alleged measures of other constructs, respectively.

The term *validity* is also used in the context of research design. An experimental study is said to be internally valid if the effect on the dependent variable can actually be attributed to the independent variable that has been manipulated, and not to some uncontrolled competing threat(s). Any study is said to be externally valid if the results are generalizable to persons and conditions other than those directly involved in the study.

In certain kinds of research there is the need for cross-validation of the findings. Regression analyses are particularly prone to "overfitting" the sample data, so whenever possible one should divide the subjects randomly into two groups, derive the regression coefficients for each of the two groups separately and then determine how well Group A's regression equation "predicts" Group B's scores on the dependent variable, and vice versa.

Example: The "mirror test" is one way of measuring obesity (look at yourself in a mirror and determine whether you're obese or not) and is generally regarded as content valid. The use of calipers to determine skin fold thickness is a more objective, but also content-valid, way of measuring obesity. It could serve as an external criterion for determining the criterion-related validity of indirect measures of obesity such as the body mass index (weight divided by the square of height). And any instrument for measuring obesity should correlate positively with variables such as caloric intake and waist circumference, but should not correlate with variables such as body temperature if those instruments are to have acceptable construct validity.

Qualitative researchers use terms such as *truth value, credibility, trustworthiness,* and *accuracy* to describe their concerns about the soundness of their data. Ways of managing threats to "internal validity" (the term is not used in the Campbell & Stanley, 1966, sense), for example, subject bias, reactive effects of the researcher, and changes in the study situation over time, are built into data collection and analysis procedures. These procedures include detailed record keeping, analytical notes accounting for personal actions and subjective

183

thoughts and impressions of the researcher, multiple approaches to verification of data, and the simultaneous collection and analysis of data to examine their adequacy and to correct inaccuracies and imbalances.

The issue of external validity, or generalizability of results, relates to sampling procedures that involve the researcher's judgment about which subject characteristics will be considered as representative of a larger population. Sampling is often theoretical rather than statistical. (*See* **Grounded Theory** and **Theoretical Sampling**.) Discussions about the evaluative criteria to apply when judging the adequacy of a qualitative study have generated a variety of considerations, a number of terms used in place of or instead of *validity*, and different stances on how closely measures of validity in qualitative and quantitative research are, or should be, parallel to each other (Brink, 1991; Fielding & Fielding, 1986; Glaser & Strauss, 1967; Homans, 1955; Kirk & Miller, 1986; LeCompte & Goetz, 1982; Leininger, 1994; Lincoln & Guba, 1985; Miles & Huberman, 1984a, 1984b; Sandelowski, 1986; Smith & Heshusius, 1986).

Variable

A variable is an operationalization of a construct.

It may be a "good" operationalization in which case the measuring instrument is said to be *valid*, or it may be a "bad," or invalid, operationalization. As the name implies, it must be possible to obtain more than one "score" on that variable; otherwise it would be a constant. Variables that produce a wide spread of scores are especially useful in research, as one of the main objectives is to study how two dimensions "covary." If the operationalizations of two constructs do not vary, or vary only slightly, then covariability cannot be properly investigated.

Variables can be classified in several different ways. There are continuous versus discrete variables (a discrete variable that has just two categories is called a dichotomy); "manifest" versus "latent" variables (the latter are the constructs themselves); nominal, ordinal, interval, and ratio variables; independent versus dependent variables; antecedent variables, extraneous variables, and mediating variables; and so on. It is the independent versus dependent distinction that is most widely discussed.

Although some authors distinguish between independent and dependent variables only within the context of experimental research, the terms apply equally well to nonexperimental research in which an independent variable is a predictor variable that is supposed to help in "explaining" the dependent (criterion) variable. However, the independent/dependent distinction breaks down completely in certain studies, for example, factor analytic studies, where all of the variables are on "equal footing" with one another, that is, none of them is regarded as any sort of cause and none is regarded as any sort of effect.

A common confusion is the labeling of a *category* of a variable as a variable. Stated political preference is a variable; Democrat, Republican, and so on are categories of the variable. Self-reported socioeconomic status is a variable; upper class, upper-middle class, and so forth are categories of that variable. Statements such as "there is a strong relationship between being a Democrat and being lower-middle class" are methodologically incorrect. Relationships hold between variables, not categories, even though it is the relative frequency of certain combinations of categories that produce those relationships. It is often easier to phrase the research question in terms of relationships between categories than in terms of relationships between variables. For example, "What is the relationship between smoking and lung cancer?" although incorrect, flows more naturally than "What is the relationship between number of cigarettes smoked and amount of lung cancer?"

Example: Although not usually regarded as such, sex is actually a construct. One operationalization of that construct is the self-reporting of one's "maleness" or "femaleness." Because sex is almost always "measured" this way, the distinction between construct and variable for such dimensions is rarely made, but really should be. Self-report of sex is clearly not the only way to operationalize that construct, and for very young children (especially babies) it is impractical, unreliable, and invalid.

Variance

The variance of a set of data for a variable is the mean of the squared deviations (differences) from the mean. It is the square of the standard deviation.

See **Standard Deviation**.

Visual Analogue Scale

A visual analogue scale is a line 100 millimeters in length (usually) on which various descriptors are located, and the subject is asked to

V

indicate a point on that line that represents his or her feeling about a particular matter.

Example: In assessing overall attitude toward abortion a researcher might use a visual analogue scale with the words "It should never be permitted under any circumstance" at one end of the scale and the words "It should always be permitted under any circumstance" at the other end of the scale. Possible scores for such a scale could range from 0 (for never) to 100 (for always).

Visual analogue scales yield data that can be treated as conceptually continuous and therefore appropriate for most traditional statistical analyses.

The advantages and disadvantages of visual analogue scales are summarized very nicely by Wewers and Lowe (1990) and by Cline, Herman, Shaw, and Morton (1992).

V

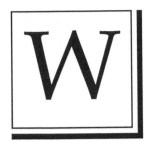

Worldview

Worldview refers to a particular social or cultural group's outlook on, and beliefs about, its world. These views could include a wide range of generally held notions about the role of the individual in society; how people ought to relate to one another; people's relationship to nature; or the role of kinship, economic, political, and religious institutions in the society and in individuals' lives. Some qualitative investigations of an ethnographic, hermeneutic, or historical nature may be particularly interested in examining the worldview of a group of people. However, it is always difficult to know what elements should be incorporated into a worldview, as all members of a group will never respond to all of the features of a worldview in precisely the same way.

W

Z

Zero-Order Correlation Coefficient

A zero-order correlation coefficient is a "Pearson r" that indicates the magnitude and direction of the "raw" linear relationship between two variables (no "partialing").

See **Partial Correlation Coefficient** and **Pearson Product-Moment Correlation Coefficient**.

REFERENCES

Aamodt, A. M. (1991). Ethnography and epistemology: Generating nursing knowledge. In J. M. Morse (Ed.), *Qualitative nursing research*. Newbury Park, CA: Sage.

Aaronson, L. S., Frey, M. A., & Boyd, C. J. (1988). Structural equation models and nursing research: Part II. *Nursing Research, 37*, 315-318.

Allen, D. (1985). Nursing research and social control: Alternative models of science that emphasize understanding and emancipation. *Image, 17*, 59-64.

Allen, D. (1986). Using philosophical and historical methodologies to understand the concept of health. In P. L. Chinn (Ed.), *Nursing research methodology*. Rockville, MD: Aspen.

Allen, D., Allman, K.K.M., & Powers, P. (1991). Feminist nursing research without gender. *Advances in Nursing Science, 13*(3), 49-58.

Allen, D., Benner, P., & Diekelmann, N. (1986). Three paradigms for nursing research: Methodological implications. In P. L. Chinn (Ed.), *Nursing research methodology*. Rockville, MD: Aspen.

Allen, D., & Whatley, M. (1986). Nursing and men's health: Some critical considerations. *Nursing Clinics of North America, 21*, 3-13.

Allison, S. E. (1993). Anna Wolf's dream: Establishment of a collegiate nursing education program. *Image, 25*, 127-131.

Armstrong, G. D. (1981). The intraclass correlation as a measure of interrater reliability of subjective judgments. *Nursing Research, 30*, 314-320.

Atkinson, P. (1992). The ethnography of a medical setting: Reading, writing, and rhetoric. *Qualitative Health Research, 2*, 451-474.

Ball, M. J., Hannah, K. J., Gerdin-Jelger, U., & Peterson, H. (1988). *Nursing informatics: Where caring and technology meet*. New York: Springer-Verlag.

Barhyte, D., Redman, B. K., & Neill, K. M. (1990). Population or sample: Design decision. *Nursing Research, 39*, 309-310.

Barkman, A., & Lunse, C. P. (1994). The effect of early ambulation on patient comfort and delayed bleeding after cardiac angiogram: A pilot study. *Heart and Lung, 23*, 112-117.

Barnum, B. J. Stevens (1994). *Nursing theory: Analysis, application, evaluation* (4th ed.). Philadelphia: J. B. Lippincott.

Baron, R. M., & Kenny, D. A. (1986). The moderator-mediator variable distinction in social psychological research: Conceptual, strategic, and statistical considerations. *Journal of Personality and Social Psychology, 51*, 1173-1182.

Barthes, R. (1984). *Mythologies*. New York: Hill & Wang.

Barthes, R. (1986). *The rustle of language*. New York: Hill & Wang.

Beck, C. T. (1992). The lived experience of postpartum depression: A phenomenological study. *Nursing Research, 41*, 166-170.

Beck, C. T. (1993). Teetering on the edge: A substantive theory of postpartum depression. *Nursing Research, 42*, 42-48.

Becker, H. S. (1958). Problems of inference and proof in participant observation. *American Sociological Review, 23*, 652-660.

Beeber, L. S. (1990). To be one of the boys: Aftershocks of the World War I nursing experience. *Advances in Nursing Science, 12*(4), 32-43.

Benner, P. (1983). Uncovering the knowledge embedded in clinical practice. *Image, 15*, 36-41.

Benner, P. (1984). *From novice to expert: Excellence and power in clinical nursing practice.* Menlo Park, CA: Addison-Wesley.

Benner, P. (1994). *Interpretive phenomenology: Embodiment, caring, and ethics in health and illness.* Thousand Oaks, CA: Sage.

Benner, P., & Tanner, C. (1987). Clinical judgment: How expert nurses use intuition. *American Journal of Nursing, 87*, 23-31.

Benner, P., & Wrubel, J. (1989). *The primacy of caring: Stress and coping in health and illness.* Menlo Park, CA: Addison-Wesley.

Berger, P., & Luckmann, T. (1967). *The social construction of reality.* Garden City, NY: Anchor.

Birnbach, N. (1993). The development of organized nursing and the Pan-American Exposition at Buffalo in 1901: Doing historical research. In P. L. Munhall & C. O. Boyd, *Nursing research: A qualitative perspective.* New York: National League for Nursing Press.

Blegen, M. A. (1993). Nurses' job satisfaction: A meta-analysis of related variables. *Nursing Research, 42*, 36-41.

Blumer, H. (1969). *Symbolic interaction: Perspective and method.* Englewood Cliffs, NJ: Prentice Hall.

Bournaki, M-C., & Germain, C. P. (1993). Esthetic knowledge in family centered nursing care of hospitalized children. *Advances in Nursing Science, 16*(2), 81-89.

Bowles, C. (1986). Measure of attitude toward menopause using the semantic differential model. *Nursing Research, 35*, 81-85.

Boyd, C. J., Frey, M. A., & Aaronson, L. S. (1988). Structural equation models and nursing research: Part I. *Nursing Research, 37*, 249-252.

Boyle, J. S. (1991). Field research: A collaborative model for practice and research. In J. M. Morse (Ed.), *Qualitative nursing research: A contemporary dialogue.* Newbury Park, CA: Sage.

Boyle, J. S. (1994). Styles of ethnography. In J. M. Morse (Ed.), *Critical issues in qualitative research methods.* Thousand Oaks, CA: Sage.

Breitmayer, B. J., Ayres, L., & Knafl, K. A. (1993). Triangulation in qualitative research: Evaluation of completeness and confirmation purposes. *Image, 25*, 237-243.

Brink, P. J. (1991). Issues in reliability and validity. In J. M. Morse (Ed.), *Qualitative nursing research: A contemporary dialogue* (rev. ed.). Newbury Park, CA: Sage.

Brink, P. J., & Wood, M. J. (1983). *Basic steps in planning nursing research, from question to proposal* (2nd ed.). Monterey, CA: Wadsworth.

Brown, J. K., Porter, L. A., & Knapp, T. R. (1993). The applicability of sequential analysis to nursing research. *Nursing Research, 42*, 280-282.

Brown, M. A., & Powell-Cope, G. M. (1991). AIDS family caregiving: Transitions through uncertainty. *Nursing Research, 40*, 338-345.

Bullough, V. L., Bullough, B., & Wu, Y-W. B. (1992). Achievement of eminent American nurses of the past: A prosopographical study. *Nursing Research, 41*, 120-124.

Bunting, S., & Campbell, J. C. (1990). Feminism and nursing: Historical perspectives. *Advances in Nursing Science, 12*(4), 11-24.

Campbell, D. T., & Fiske, D. W. (1959). Convergent and discriminant validation by the multitrait-multimethod matrix. *Psychological Bulletin, 56*, 81-105.

Campbell, D. T., & Stanley, J. C. (1966). *Experimental and quasi-experimental designs for research.* Chicago: Rand McNally.

Campbell, J. C., & Bunting, S. (1991). Voices and paradigms: Perspectives on critical and feminist theory in nursing. *Advances in Nursing Science, 13*(3), 1-15.

Carey, M. A. (1994). The group effect in focus groups: Planning, implementing, and interpreting focus group research. In J. M. Morse (Ed.), *Critical issues in qualitative research.* Thousand Oaks, CA: Sage.

Carey, M. A., & Smith, M. W. (1994). Capturing the group effect in focus groups: A special concern in analysis. *Qualitative Health Research, 14,* 123-127.

Carmines, E. G., & Zeller, R. A. (1979). *Reliability and validity assessment.* Beverly Hills, CA: Sage.

Caroline, H. A., & Bernhard, L. A. (1994). Health care dilemmas for women with serious mental illness. *Advances in Nursing Science, 16*(3), 78-88.

Carper, B. A. (1978). Fundamental patterns of knowing in nursing. *Advances in Nursing Science, 1*(1), 13-23.

Carter, E., & Fielding, J. for the New York State Nurses Association (NYSNA) Council on Nursing Research and the Foundation of the New York State Nurses Association. (1988). *Professionalization of nursing in New York state: Oral history interviews with six leaders who helped to advance the mission of NYSNA.* Guilderland, NY: New York State Nurses Association.

Chenitz, W. C., & Swanson, J. M. (1986). *From practice to grounded theory: Qualitative research in nursing.* Menlo Park, CA: Addison-Wesley.

Chinn, P. L. (1994). Developing a method for aesthetic knowing in nursing. In P. L. Chinn & J. Watson (Eds.), *Art and aesthetics in nursing.* New York: National League for Nursing Press.

Chinn, P. L., & Kramer, M. K. (1995). *Theory and nursing: A systematic approach* (4th ed.). St. Louis: C. V. Mosby.

Chinn, P. L., & Watson, J. (Eds.). (1994). *Art and aesthetics in nursing.* New York: National League for Nursing Press.

Christman, N. J., & Johnson, J. E. (1981). The importance of research in nursing. In Y. M. Williamson (Ed.), *Research methodology and its application to nursing.* New York: John Wiley.

Cicourel, A. V. (1968). *The social organization of juvenile justice.* New York: John Wiley.

Cline, M., Herman, J., Shaw, E. R., & Morton, R. D. (1992). Standardization of the visual analogue scale. *Nursing Research, 41,* 378-380.

Cohen, J. (1988). *Statistical power analysis for the behavioral sciences* (2nd ed.). Hillsdale, NJ: Lawrence Erlbaum.

Cohen, J., & Cohen, P. (1983). *Applied multiple regression/correlation analysis for the behavioral sciences* (2nd ed.). Hillsdale, NJ: Lawrence Erlbaum.

Cohen, M. Z., & Omery, A. (1994). Schools of phenomenology: Implications for research. In J. M. Morse (Ed.), *Critical issues in qualitative research methods.* Thousand Oaks, CA: Sage.

Connelly, L. M., Keele, B. S., Kleinbeck, S.V.M., Schneider, J. K., & Cobb, A. K. (1993). A place to be yourself: Empowerment from the client's perspective. *Image, 25,* 297-303.

Cook, T. D., & Campbell, D. T. (1979). *Quasi-experimentation: Design and analysis issues for field settings.* Chicago: Rand McNally.

Cramer, S. (1992). The nature of history: Meditations on Clio's craft. *Nursing Research, 41,* 4-7.

Criddle, L. (1993). Healing from surgery: A phenomenological study. *Image, 25,* 208-213.

Cronbach, L. J. (1951). Coefficient alpha and the internal structure of tests. *Psychometrika, 16,* 297-334.

Davis, G. C. (1992). The meaning of pain management: A concept analysis. *Advances in Nursing Science, 15*(1), 77-86.

DeKeyser, F. G., & Pugh, L. C. (1990). Assessment of the reliability and validity of biochemical measures. *Nursing Research, 39,* 314-317.

DeMarco, R., Campbell, J., & Wuest, J. (1993). Feminist critique: Searching for meaning in research. *Advances in Nursing Science, 16*(2), 26-38.

Denzin, N. K. (1989). *Interpretive biography.* Newbury Park, CA: Sage.

Denzin, N. K. (1994). The art and politics of interpretation. In N. K. Denzin & Y. S. Lincoln (Eds.), *Handbook of qualitative research.* Thousand Oaks, CA: Sage.

Derrida, J. (1981). *Positions.* Chicago: University of Chicago Press.

Diekelmann, N. L. (1992). Learning-as-testing: A Heideggerian hermeneutical analysis of the lived experiences of students and teachers in nursing. *Advances in Nursing Science, 14*(3), 72-83.

Ditton, J. (1980). *The view from Goffman.* London: Macmillan.

Dombeck, M.-T. B. (1991). *Dreams and professional personhood: The contexts of dream telling and dream interpretation among American psychotherapists.* Albany: State University of New York Press.

Donahue, M. P. (1983). Isabel Maitland Stewart's philosophy of education. *Nursing Research, 32,* 140-146.

Donahue, M. P. (1985). *Nursing: The finest art. An illustrated history.* St. Louis: C. V. Mosby.

Donaldson, S. K., & Crowley, D. M. (1978). The discipline of nursing. *Nursing Outlook, 26,* 113-120.

Douglass, B., & Moustakas, C. (1985). Heuristic inquiry: The internal search to know. *Journal of Humanistic Psychology, 25*(3), 39-55.

Downs, F. S. (1979). Clinical and theoretical research. In F. S. Downs & J. W. Fleming (Eds.), *Issues in nursing research.* New York: Appleton-Century-Crofts.

Drew, N. (1993). Reenactment interviewing: A methodology for phenomenological research. *Image, 25,* 345-351.

Drummond, J. E., Wiebe, C. F., & Elliott, M. R. (1994). Maternal understanding of infant crying: What does a negative case tell us? *Qualitative Health Research, 4,* 208-223.

Dubin, R. (1978). *Theory building.* New York: Free Press.

Engstrom, J. L. (1988). Assessment of the reliability of physical measures. *Research in Nursing & Health, 11,* 383-389.

Eysenck, H. J. (1978). An exercise in mega-silliness. *American Psychologist, 33,* 517.

Fawcett, J. (1995). *Analysis and evaluation of conceptual models of nursing* (3rd ed.). Philadelphia: F. A. Davis.

Fay, B. (1987). *Critical social science.* Ithaca, NY: Cornell University Press.

Ferketich, S., & Verran, J. (1986). Exploratory data analysis: Introduction. *Western Journal of Nursing Research, 8,* 464-466.

Field, P. A. (1991). Doing fieldwork in your own culture. In J. M. Morse (Ed.), *Qualitative nursing research: A contemporary dialogue.* Newbury Park, CA: Sage.

Field, P. A., & Morse, J. M. (1985). *Nursing research: The application of qualitative approaches.* Rockville, MD: Aspen.

Fielding, N. G., & Fielding, J. L. (1986). *Linking data.* Beverly Hills, CA: Sage.

Fielding, N. G., & Lee, R. M. (1991). *Using computers in qualitative research.* Newbury Park, CA: Sage.

Finney, J. W., Mitchell, R. E., Cronkhite, R. C., & Moos, R. H. (1984). Methodological issues in estimating main and interactive effects: Examples from coping, social support and stress field. *Journal of Health and Social Behavior, 25,* 85-98.

Fitzpatrick, J. J., & Whall, A. L. (1989). *Conceptual models of nursing* (2nd ed.). Norwalk, CT: Appleton & Lange.

Floyd, J. A. (1983). Research using Rogers' conceptual system: Development of a testable theorem. *Advances in Nursing Science, 5*(2), 37-48.

Floyd, J. A. (1993). Systematic sampling: Theory and clinical methods. *Nursing Research, 42,* 290-293.

Fonow, M. M., & Cook, J. A. (1991). *Beyond methodology: Feminist scholarship as lived research.* Bloomington: Indiana University Press.

Foucault, M. (1961). *Madness and civilization.* London: Tavistock, 1971.

Foucault, M. (1963). *The birth of the clinic.* London: Tavistock, 1973.

Foucault, M. (1966). *The order of things.* London: Tavistock, 1974.

Foucault, M. (1969). *The archaeology of knowledge.* London: Tavistock, 1974.

Foucault, M. (1975). *Discipline and punish.* London: Tavistock, 1977.

Foucault, M. (1976). *The history of sexuality.* London: Tavistock, 1979.

Fry, S. T. (1992). Neglect of philosophical inquiry in nursing: Cause and effect. In J. F. Kikuchi & H. Simmons (Eds.), *Philosophic inquiry in nursing.* Newbury Park, CA: Sage.

Gadamer, H. G. (1976). *Philosophical hermeneutics.* Berkeley: University of California Press.

Garfinkel, H. (1967). *Studies in ethnomethodology.* Englewood Cliffs, NJ: Prentice Hall.

Geertz, C. (1973). *The interpretation of cultures: Selected essays.* New York: Basic Books.

Geertz, C. (1983). *Local knowledge: Further essays in interpretive anthropology.* New York: Basic Books.

Gilligan, C. (1982). *In a different voice.* Cambridge, MA: Harvard University Press.

Glaser, B. G. (1978). *Theoretical sensitivity.* Mill Valley, CA: Sociology Press.

Glaser, B. G. (1992). *Emergence versus forcing: Basics of grounded theory analysis.* Mill Valley, CA: Sociology Press.

Glaser, B. G., & Strauss, A. L. (1965). *Awareness of dying.* Chicago: Aldine.

Glaser, B. G., & Strauss, A. L. (1967). *The discovery of grounded theory: Strategies for qualitative research.* Chicago: Aldine.

Glaser, B. G., & Strauss, A. L. (1968). *Time for dying.* Chicago: Aldine.

Glaser, B. G., & Strauss, A. L. (1971). *Status passage: A formal theory.* Chicago: Aldine.

Glass, G. V (1976). Primary, secondary, and meta-analysis of research. *Educational Researcher, 5,* 3-8.

Goffman, E. (1959). *The presentation of self in everyday life.* Garden City, NY: Doubleday Anchor.

Goffman, E. (1961). *Asylums.* Harmondsworth, UK: Penguin.

Goffman, E. (1963). *Behavior in public places: Notes on the social organization of gatherings.* New York: Free Press.

Goffman, E. (1967). *Interaction ritual: Essays in face-to-face behavior.* Chicago: Aldine.

Goffman, E. (1971). *Relations in public: Microstudies of the public order.* New York: Basic Books.

Goode, C. J., Titler, M., Rakel, B., Ones, D. Z., Kleiber, C., Small, S., & Triolo, P. K. (1991). A meta-analysis of effects of heparin flush and saline flush: Quality and cost implications. *Nursing Research, 40,* 324-330.

Goodwin, L. D., & Goodwin, W. L. (1984). Qualitative *vs.* quantitative research or qualitative *and* quantitative research? *Nursing Research, 33,* 378-380.

Gulick, E. E. (1994). Social support among persons with multiple sclerosis. *Research in Nursing and Health, 17,* 195-206.

Guttman, L. (1941). The quantification of a class of attributes: A theory and method for scale construction. In P. Horst (Ed.), *The prediction of personal adjustment.* New York: Social Science Research Council.

Habermas, J. (1971). *Knowledge and human interests.* Boston: Beacon.

Hall, J. M. (1994a). How lesbians recognize and respond to alcohol problems: A theoretical model of problematization. *Advances in Nursing Science, 16*(3), 46-63.

Hall, J. M. (1994b). Lesbians recovering from alcohol problems: An ethnographic study of health care experiences. *Nursing Research, 43,* 238-244.

Hall, J. M., & Stevens, P. E. (1991). Rigor in feminist research. *Advances in Nursing Science, 13*(3), 16-29.

Halpern, E. S. (1983). *Auditing naturalistic inquiries: The development and application of a model.* Unpublished doctoral dissertation, Indiana University.

Hamilton, D. B. (1993). The idea of history and the history of ideas. *Image, 25,* 45-48.

Hannah, K. J., Ball, M. J., & Edwards, M.J.A. (1994). *Introduction to nursing informatics.* New York: Springer-Verlag.

Harding, S. (1987). Conclusion: Epistemological questions. In S. Harding (Ed.), *Feminism and methodology: Social science issues.* Bloomington: Indiana University Press.

Hardy, M. E. (1978). Perspectives on nursing theory. *Advances in Nursing Science, 1*(1), 37-48.

Harris, R. J. (1985). *A primer of multivariate statistics* (2nd ed.). New York: Academic Press.

Hawkes, T. (1977). *Structuralism and semiotics.* Berkeley: University of California Press.

Hays, B. J., Norris, J., Martin, K. S., & Androwich, I. (1994). Informatics issues for nursing's future. *Advances in Nursing Science, 16*(4), 71-81.

Hebdige, D. (1979). *Subculture: The meaning of style.* London: Methuen.

Hedin, B. A. (1986). A case study of oppressed group behavior in nurses. *Image, 18,* 53-57.

Heidegger, M. (1962). *Being and time.* New York: Harper & Row.

Heidegger, M. (1975). *Poetry, language and thought.* New York: Harper & Row.

Held, D. (1980). *Introduction to critical theory.* Berkeley: University of California Press.

Hess, B. (1990). Beyond dichotomy: Drawing distinctions and embracing differences. *Sociological Forum, 5,* 75-94.

Hill, M. R. (1993). *Archival strategies and techniques.* Newbury Park, CA: Sage.

Hiraki, A. (1992). Tradition, rationality, and power in introductory nursing textbooks: A critical hermeneutics study. *Advances in Nursing Science, 14*(3), 1-12.

Hitchcock, J. M., & Wilson, H. S. (1992). Personal risking: Lesbian self-disclosure of sexual orientation to professional health care providers. *Nursing Research, 41,* 178-183.

Hodder, I. (1994). The interpretation of documents and material culture. In N. K. Denzin & Y. S. Lincoln (Eds.), *Handbook of qualitative research.* Thousand Oaks, CA: Sage.

Hogan, N., & DeSantis, L. (1992). Adolescent sibling bereavement: An ongoing attachment. *Qualitative Health Research, 2,* 159-177.

Holm, K. (1983). Single subject research. *Nursing Research, 32,* 253-255.

Holsti, O. R. (1969). *Content analysis for the social sciences and humanities.* Reading, MA: Addison-Wesley.

Homans, G. C. (1955). *The human group.* New York: Harcourt, Brace.

Howell, S. L. (1994). A theoretical model for caring for women with chronic nonmalignant pain. *Qualitative Health Research, 4*, 94-122.

Hoy, D. C. (1986). *Foucault: A critical reader.* New York: Basil Blackwell.

Huberman, A. M., & Miles, M. B. (1994). Data management and analysis methods. In N. K. Denzin & Y. S. Lincoln (Eds.), *Handbook of qualitative research.* Thousand Oaks, CA: Sage.

Hughes, C. C. (1992). "Ethnography": What's in a word—Process? Product? Promise? *Qualitative Health Research, 2*, 439-450.

Hughes, L. (1990). Professionalizing domesticity: A synthesis of selected nursing historiography. *Advances in Nursing Science, 12*(4), 25-31.

Husserl, E. (1965). *Phenomenology and the crisis of philosophy.* New York: Harper & Row.

Husserl, E. (1970). *The crisis of European sciences and transcendental phenomenology.* Evanston, IL: Northwestern University Press.

Husserl, E. (1977). *Cartesian meditations: An introduction to phenomenology.* The Hague, The Netherlands: Martinus Nijhoff.

Ihde, D. (1971). *Hermeneutic phenomenology. The philosophy of Paul Ricoeur.* Evanston, IL: Northwestern University Press.

Jacobsen, B. S. (1981). Know thy data. *Nursing Research, 30*, 254-255.

Jacobson, G. (1994). The meaning of stressful life experiences in nine- to eleven-year-old children: A phenomenological study. *Nursing Research, 43*, 95-99.

Janke, J. (1994). Development of the breast-feeding attrition prediction tool. *Nursing Research, 43*, 100-104.

Jaspers, K. (1968). The phenomenological approach in psychopathology. *British Journal of Psychiatry, 114*, 1313-1323.

Johnson, J. L., Ratner, P. A., Bottorff, J. L., & Hayduk, L. A. (1993). An exploration of Pender's Health Promotion Model using LISREL. *Nursing Research, 42*, 132-138.

Kaplan, A. (1964). *The conduct of inquiry.* New York: Thomas Y. Crowell.

Kauffman, K. S. (1994). The insider/outsider dilemma: Field experience of a white researcher "getting in" a poor black community. *Nursing Research, 43*, 179-183.

Kidd, P. S. (1992). Skeletons in the closet: The ICU nurse as novice field worker in the ICU. *Qualitative Health Research, 2*, 497-503.

Kiecolt, K. J., & Nathan, L. E. (1985). *Secondary analysis of survey data.* Newbury Park, CA: Sage.

Kikuchi, J. F. (1992). Nursing questions that science cannot answer. In J. F. Kikuchi & H. Simmons (Eds.), *Philosophic inquiry in nursing.* Newbury Park, CA: Sage.

Kikuchi, J. F., & Simmons, H. (Eds.). (1992). *Philosophic inquiry in nursing.* Newbury Park, CA: Sage.

Kimchi, J., Polivka, B., & Stevenson, J. S. (1991). Triangulation: Operational definitions. *Nursing Research, 40*, 364-366.

Kincheloe, J. L., & McLaren, P. L. (1994). Rethinking critical theory and qualitative research. In N. K. Denzin & Y. S. Lincoln (Eds.), *Handbook of qualitative research.* Thousand Oaks, CA: Sage.

King, I. (1971). *Toward a theory of nursing.* New York: John Wiley.

King, I. (1981). *A theory for nursing: Systems, concepts, process.* New York: John Wiley.

King, K. B., Porter, L. A., Norsen, L. H., & Reis, H. T. (1992). Patient perceptions of quality of life after coronary artery surgery: Was it worth it? *Research in Nursing and Health, 15*, 327-334.

Kingry, M. J., Tiedje, L. B., & Friedman, L. L. (1990). Focus groups: A research technique for nursing. *Nursing Research, 39*, 124-125.

Kirk, J., & Miller, M. L. (1986). *Reliability and validity in qualitative research.* Beverly Hills, CA: Sage.

Kleinbaum, D. G., Kupper, L. L., & Morgenstern, H. (1982). *Epidemiologic research: Principles and quantitative methods.* Belmont, CA: Wadsworth.

Kleinman, A. (1992). Local worlds of suffering: An interpersonal focus for ethnographies of illness experience. *Qualitative Health Research, 2,* 127-134.

Knapp, T. R. (1985). Validity, reliability, and neither. *Nursing Research, 34,* 189-192.

Knapp, T. R. (1990). Treating ordinal scales as interval scales: An attempt to resolve the controversy. *Nursing Research, 39,* 121-123.

Knapp, T. R. (1991). Coefficient alpha: Conceptualizations and anomalies. *Research in Nursing and Health, 14,* 457-460.

Knapp, T. R. (1993). Treating ordinal scales as ordinal scales. *Nursing Research, 42,* 184-186.

Knapp, T. R. (1994). Regression analyses: What to report. *Nursing Research, 43,* 187-189.

Kolcaba, K. Y. (1991). A taxonomic structure for the concept comfort. *Image, 23,* 237-240.

Kondora, L. L. (1993). A Heideggerian hermeneutical analysis of survivors of incest. *Image, 25,* 11-16.

Krippendorff, K. (1980). *Content analysis.* Beverly Hills, CA: Sage.

Krueger, R. A. (1994). *Focus groups: A practical guide for applied research* (2nd ed.). Thousand Oaks, CA: Sage.

Krywanio, M. L. (1994). Meta-analysis of physiological outcomes of hospital-based infant intervention programs. *Nursing Research, 43,* 133-137.

Kuhn, T. S. (1970). *The structure of scientific revolutions* (2nd ed.). Chicago: University of Chicago Press.

Kuhn, T. S. (1977). *The essential tension.* Chicago: University of Chicago Press.

Lamendola, F. P., & Newman, M. A. (1994). The paradox of HIV/AIDS as expanding consciousness. *Advances in Nursing Science, 16*(3), 13-21.

Lancaster, W., & Lancaster, J. (1992). Models and model building in nursing. In L. H. Nicoll (Ed.), *Perspectives on nursing theory* (2nd ed.). New York: J. B. Lippincott.

Last, J. M. (Ed.). (1988). *A dictionary of epidemiology* (2nd ed.). New York: Oxford University Press.

Lather, P. (1991). *Getting smart: Feminist research and pedagogy with/in the postmodern.* New York: Routledge.

Lauden, L. (1977). *Progress and its problems: Toward a theory of scientific growth.* Berkeley: University of California Press.

Lauterbach, S. S. (1993). In another world: A phenomenological perspective and discovery of meaning in mothers' experience with death of a wished-for baby: Doing phenomenology. In P. L. Munhall & C. O. Boyd (Eds.), *Nursing research: A qualitative perspective* (2nd ed.). New York: National League for Nursing Press.

LeCompte, M. D., & Goetz, J. P. (1982). Problems of reliability and validity in ethnographic research. *Review of Educational Research, 52,* 31-60.

Leininger, M. M. (Ed.). (1985). *Qualitative research methods in nursing.* Orlando, FL: Grune & Stratton.

Leininger, M. M. (Ed.). (1991). *Culture care diversity and universality: A theory of nursing.* New York: National League for Nursing.

Leininger, M. M. (1994). Evaluation criteria and critique of qualitative research studies. In J. M. Morse (Ed.), *Critical issues in qualitative research methods.* Thousand Oaks, CA: Sage.

Likert, R. (1932). A technique for the measurement of attitudes. *Archives of Psychology, 22,* 5-55.

Lincoln, Y. S., & Guba, E. G. (1985). *Naturalistic inquiry.* Beverly Hills, CA: Sage.

Lindeman, C. (1975). Delphi survey of priorities in clinical nursing research. *Nursing Research, 24,* 434-444.

Lindley, P., & Walker, S. N. (1993). Theoretical and methodological differentiation of moderation and mediation. *Nursing Research, 42,* 276-279.

Lipson, J. G. (1991a). Afghan refugee health: Some findings and suggestions. *Qualitative Health Research, 1,* 349-369.

Lipson, J. G. (1991b). The use of self in ethnographic research. In J. M. Morse (Ed.), *Qualitative nursing research: A contemporary dialogue.* Newbury Park, CA: Sage.

Lucas, M. D., Atwood, J. R., & Hagaman, R. (1993). Replication and validation of Anticipated Turnover Model for urban registered nurses. *Nursing Research, 42,* 184-186.

Lusk, S. L., Ronis, D. L., Kerr, M. J., & Atwood, J. R. (1994). Test of the Health Promotion Model as a causal model of workers' use of hearing protection. *Nursing Research, 43,* 151-157.

MacAndrew, C., & Edgerton, R. (1969). *Drunken comportment.* Chicago: Aldine.

MacLeod, J. (1987). *Ain't no makin' it: Leveled aspirations in a low-income neighborhood.* Boulder, CO: Westview.

MacPherson, K. I. (1983). Feminist methods: A new paradigm for nursing research. *Advances in Nursing Science, 5*(1), 17-26.

MacPherson, K. I. (1992). Cardiovascular disease in women and noncontraceptive use of hormones: A feminist analysis. *Advances in Nursing Science, 14*(4), 34-49.

Magilvy, J. K., Congdon, J. G., & Martinez, R. (1994). Circles of care: Home care and community support for rural older adults. *Advances in Nursing Science, 16*(3), 22-33.

Malinowski, B. (1922). *Argonauts of the Western Pacific.* London: Routledge.

Manning, P. K. (1987). *Semiotics and fieldwork.* Newbury Park, CA: Sage.

Manning, P. K., & Cullum-Swan, B. (1994). Narrative, content, and semiotic analysis. In N. K. Denzin & Y. S. Lincoln (Eds.), *Handbook of qualitative research,* Thousand Oaks, CA: Sage.

Marascuilo, L. A., & Levin, J. R. (1983). *Multivariate statistics in the social sciences.* Pacific Grove, CA: Brooks/Cole.

Marriner-Tomey, A. (1994). *Nursing theorists and their work* (3rd ed.). St. Louis: C. V. Mosby.

McArt, E. W., & McDougal, L. W. (1985). Secondary data analysis: A new approach to nursing research. *Image, 17,* 54-57.

McCall, W. A. (1939). *Measurement.* New York: Macmillan.

McHugh, P. (1968). *Defining the situation.* Indianapolis, IN: Bobbs-Merrill.

McKillip, J. (1987). *Need analysis: Tools for the human services and education.* Beverly Hills, CA: Sage.

McLain, B. R. (1988). Collaborative practice: A critical theory perspective. *Research in Nursing and Health, 11,* 391-398.

McLaughlin, F. E., & Marascuilo, L. A. (1990). *Advanced nursing and health care research: Quantification approaches.* Philadelphia: W. B. Saunders.

Mead, G. H. (1934). *Mind, self and society.* Chicago: University of Chicago Press.

Mead, G. H. (1938). *The philosophy of the act.* Chicago: University of Chicago Press.

Mead, G. H. (1959). *The philosophy of the present.* Seattle, WA: Open Court.

Mehan, H., & Wood, H. (1975). *The reality of ethnomethodology.* New York: John Wiley.

Meleis, A. I. (1991). *Theoretical nursing: Development and progress* (2nd ed.). Philadelphia: J. B. Lippincott.

Melosh, B. (1982). *The physician's hand.* Philadelphia: Temple University Press.

Meltzer, B. N., Petras, J. W., & Reynolds, L. T. (1975). *Symbolic interactionism.* London: Routledge & Kegan Paul.

Merleau-Ponty, M. (1962). *Phenomenology of perception.* London: Routledge & Kegan Paul.

Merleau-Ponty, M. (1964). *The primacy of perception.* Evanston, IL: Northwestern University Press.

Miles, M. B., & Huberman, A. M. (1984a). Drawing valid meaning from qualitative data: Toward a shared craft. *Educational Researcher, 13,* 20-30.

Miles, M. B., & Huberman, A. M. (1984b). *Qualitative data analysis.* Beverly Hills, CA: Sage.

Miles, M. B., & Huberman, A. M. (1994). *Qualitative data analysis: An expanded source book* (2nd ed.). Newbury Park, CA: Sage.

Miller, M. P. (1991). Factors promoting wellness in the aged person: An ethnographic study. *Advances in Nursing Science, 13*(4), 38-51.

Moccia, P. (1985). A further investigation of "Dialectical thinking as a means of understanding systems-in-development: Relevance to Rogers's principles." *Advances in Nursing Science, 7*(4), 33-38.

Moccia, P. (1986). The dialectic as method. In P. L. Chinn (Ed.), *Nursing research methodology.* Rockville, MD: Aspen.

Montgomery, C. (1994). Swimming upstream: The strengths of women who survive homelessness. *Advances in Nursing Science, 16*(3), 34-45.

Morgan, D. L. (Ed.). (1993). *Successful focus groups: Advancing the state of the art.* Newbury Park, CA: Sage.

Morgan, D. L., & Zhao, P. Z. (1993). The doctor-caregiver relationship: Managing the care of family members with Alzheimer's Disease. *Qualitative Health Research, 3,* 133-164.

Morse, J. M. (1991a). Approaches to qualitative-quantitative methodological triangulation. *Nursing Research, 40,* 120-122.

Morse, J. M. (1991b). Qualitative nursing research: A free-for-all? In J. M. Morse (Ed.), *Qualitative nursing research: A contemporary dialogue.* Newbury Park, CA: Sage.

Morse, J. M. (1991c). *Qualitative nursing research: A contemporary dialogue.* Newbury Park, CA: Sage.

Morse, J. M. (Ed.). (1994). *Critical issues in qualitative research methods.* Thousand Oaks, CA: Sage.

Morse, J. M., & Johnson, J. L. (1991). *The illness experience: Dimensions of suffering.* Newbury Park, CA: Sage.

Moustakas, C. (1967). Heuristic research. In J.F.T. Bugental (Ed.), *Challenges of humanistic psychology.* New York: McGraw-Hill.

Moustakas, C. (1990). *Heuristic research: Design, methodology, and applications.* Newbury Park, CA: Sage.

Muecke, M. A. (1994). On the evaluation of ethnographies. In J. M. Morse (Ed.), *Critical issues in qualitative research methods.* Thousand Oaks, CA: Sage.

Müller, M. E., & Dzurec, L. C. (1993). The power of the name. *Advances in Nursing Science, 15*(3), 15-22.

Mullins, N. C. (1973). *Theories and theory groups in contemporary American sociology.* New York: Harper & Row.

Munhall, P. L. (1994). *Revisioning phenomenology: Nursing and health science research*. New York: National League for Nursing Press.

Munhall, P. L., & Boyd, C. O. (1993). *Nursing research: A qualitative perspective* (2nd ed.). New York: National League for Nursing Press.

Munhall, P. L., & Oiler, C. J. (1986). *Nursing research: A qualitative perspective*. Norwalk, CT: Appleton-Century-Crofts.

Munro, B. H., & Page, E. B. (1993). *Statistical methods for health care research* (2nd ed.). Philadelphia: J. B. Lippincott.

Narsavage, G. L., & Weaver, T. E. (1994). Physiologic status, coping, and hardiness as predictors of outcomes in chronic obstructive pulmonary disease. *Nursing Research, 43*, 90-94.

Natanson, M. (1973). *Edmund Husserl: Philosopher of infinite tasks*. Evanston, IL: Northwestern University Press.

Newman, M. A. (1979). *Theory development in nursing*. Philadelphia: F. A. Davis.

Newman, M. A. (1986). *Health as expanding consciousness*. St. Louis: C. V. Mosby.

Nielsen, J. M. (1990). *Feminist research methods: Exemplary readings in the social sciences*. Boulder, CO: Westview.

Nokes, K. M., Wheeler, K., & Kendrew, J. (1994). Development of an HIV assessment tool. *Image, 26*, 133-138.

Norbeck, J. S. (1981). Social support: A model for clinical research and application. *Advances in Nursing Science, 3*(4), 43-59.

Norman, E., & Elfried, S. (1993). The angels of Bataan. *Image, 25*, 121-126.

Norman, E. M. (1992). After the casualties: Vietnam nurses' identities and career decisions. *Nursing Research, 41*, 110-113.

Nunnally, J. C., & Bernstein, I. H. (1994). *Psychometric theory* (3rd ed.). New York: McGraw-Hill.

O'Flynn, A. (1982). Meta-analysis. *Nursing Research, 31*, 314-316.

Olesen, V. (1994). Feminisms and models of qualitative research. In N. K. Denzin & Y. S. Lincoln (Eds.), *Handbook of qualitative research*. Thousand Oaks, CA: Sage.

Olson, C. T. (1993). *The life of illness: One woman's journey*. Albany: State University of New York Press.

Opie, A. (1992). Qualitative research, appropriation of the "other," and empowerment. *Feminist Review, 40*, 52-69.

Orlando, I. J. (1961). *The dynamic nurse-patient relationship*. New York: G. P. Putnam.

Osgood, C. E., Suci, G. H., & Tannenbaum, P. H. (1957). *The measurement of meaning*. Urbana: University of Illinois Press.

O'Sullivan, A. L., & Jacobsen, B. (1992). A randomized trial of a health care program for first-time adolescent mothers and their infants. *Nursing Research, 41*, 210-215.

Padilla, R. V. (1993). Using dialogical research methods in group interviews. In D. L. Morgan (Ed.), *Successful focus groups: Advancing the state of the art*. Newbury Park, CA: Sage.

Palmer, R. E. (1969). *Hermeneutics*. Evanston, IL: Northwestern University Press.

Parse, R. R. (1981). *Man-living-health: A theory of nursing*. New York: John Wiley.

Parse, R. R. (1992). Human becoming: Parse's theory of nursing. *Nursing Science Quarterly, 5*, 35-42.

Parse, R. R., Coyne, A. B., & Smith, M. J. (1985). *Nursing research: Qualitative methods*. Bowie, MD: Brady.

Paterson, B., & Bramadat, I. J. (1992). Use of the preinterview in oral history. *Qualitative Health Research, 2*, 99-115.

Pedhazur, E. J. (1982). *Multiple regression in behavioral research* (2nd ed.). New York: Holt, Rinehart & Winston.

Peplau, H. E. (1952). *Interpersonal relations in nursing.* New York: G. P. Putnam.

Peplau, H. E. (1992). Interpersonal relations: A theoretical framework for application in nursing practice. *Nursing Science Quarterly, 5,* 13-18.

Pohl, J. M., & Boyd, C. J. (1993). Ageism within feminism. *Image, 25,* 199-203.

Polit, D. F., & Hungler, B. P. (1991). *Nursing research: Principles and methods* (4th ed.). Philadelphia: J. B. Lippincott.

Polivka, B. J., & Nickel, J. T. (1992). Case-control design: An appropriate strategy for nursing research. *Nursing Research, 41,* 250-253.

Porter, E. J. (1994). Older widows' experience of living alone at home. *Image, 26,* 19-24.

Poslusny, S. M. (1989). Feminist friendship: Isabel Hampton Robb, Lavinia Lloyd Dock, and Mary Adelaide Nutting. *Image, 21,* 64-68.

Powers, B. A. (1987). Taking sides: A response to Goodwin and Goodwin. *Nursing Research, 36,* 122-126.

Powers, B. A. (1988a). Social networks, social support, and elderly institutionalized people. *Advances in Nursing Science, 10*(2), 40-58.

Powers, B. A. (1988b). Self-perceived health of elderly institutionalized people. *Journal of Cross-Cultural Gerontology, 3,* 299-321.

Powers, B. A. (1991). The meaning of nursing home friendships. *Advances in Nursing Science, 14*(2), 42-58.

Powers, B. A. (1992). The roles staff play in the social networks of elderly institutionalized people. *Social Science and Medicine, 34,* 1335-1343.

Prescott, P. A., & Soeken, K. L. (1989). The potential uses of pilot work. *Nursing Research, 38,* 60-62.

Puntillo, K., & Weiss, S. J. (1994). Pain: Its mediators and associated morbidity in critically ill cardiovascular surgical patients. *Nursing Research, 43,* 31-36.

Putnam, H. (1962). What theories are not. In E. Nagel, P. Suppes, & A. Tarski (Eds.), *Logic, methodology, and philosophy of science. Proceedings of the 1960 International Congress.* Stanford, CA: Stanford University Press.

Rabinow, P. (1984). *The Foucault reader.* New York: Pantheon.

Rather, M. L. (1992). "Nursing as a way of thinking": Heideggerian hermeneutical analysis of the lived experience of the returning RN. *Research in Nursing and Health, 15,* 47-55.

Ray, M. A. (1994). The richness of phenomenology: Philosophic, theoretic, and methodologic concerns. In J. M. Morse (Ed.), *Critical issues in qualitative research methods.* Thousand Oaks, CA: Sage.

Reed, P. G. (1991). Self-transcendence and mental health in oldest-old adults. *Nursing Research, 40,* 5-11.

Reeder, H. P. (1986). *The theory and practice of Husserl's phenomenology.* Lanham, MD: University Press of America.

Reinhard, S. C. (1994). Living with mental illness: Effects of professional support and personal control on caregiver burden. *Research in Nursing and Health, 17,* 99-110.

Rempusheski, V. F. (1988). Caring for self and others: Second generation Polish American elders in an ethnic club. *Journal of Cross-Cultural Gerontology, 3,* 223-271.

Rew, L., Bechtel, D., & Sapp, A. (1993). Self-as-instrument in qualitative research. *Nursing Research, 42,* 300-301.

Reynolds, N. R., Timmerman, G., Anderson, J., & Stevenson, J. S. (1992). Meta-analysis for descriptive research. *Research in Nursing and Health, 15,* 467-475.

Richards, L., & Richards, T. (1991). Computing in qualitative analysis: A healthy development? *Qualitative Health Research, 1,* 234-262.

Richards, T. J., & Richards, L. (1994). Using computers in qualitative research. In N. K. Denzin & Y. S. Lincoln (Eds.), *Handbook of qualitative research.* Thousand Oaks, CA: Sage.

Rickman, H. P. (1976). *Dilthey: Selected writings.* New York: Cambridge University Press.

Ricoeur, P. (1981). *Hermeneutics and the human sciences.* New York: Cambridge University Press.

Rizzuto, C., Bostrom, J., Suter, W. N., & Chenitz, W. C. (1994). Predictors of nurses' involvement in research activities. *Western Journal of Nursing Research, 16,* 193-204.

Robb, S. S. (1981). Nurse involvement in institutional review boards: The service setting perspective. *Nursing Research, 30,* 27-29.

Rodgers, B. L., & Cowles, K. V. (1993). The qualitative research audit trail: A complex collection of documentation. *Research in Nursing and Health, 16,* 219-226.

Rose, A. M. (Ed.). (1962). *Human behavior and social processes.* London: Routledge & Kegan Paul.

Rosengren, K. E. (1981). *Advances in content analysis.* Beverly Hills, CA: Sage.

Roy, C. (1984). *Introduction to nursing: An adaptation model* (2nd ed.). Englewood Cliffs, NJ: Prentice Hall.

Roy, C., & Roberts, S. (1981). *Theory construction in nursing: An adaptation model.* Englewood Cliffs, NJ: Prentice Hall.

Ryan, N. M. (1983). The epidemiological method of building causal inference. *Advances in Nursing Science, 5*(2), 73-81.

Saint-Germain, M. A., Bassford, T. L., & Montano, G. (1993). Surveys and focus groups in health research with older Hispanic women. *Qualitative Health Research, 3,* 341-367.

Sandelowski, M. (1986). The problem of rigor in qualitative research. *Advances in Nursing Science, 8*(3), 27-37.

Sandelowski, M. (1993). Rigor or rigor mortis: The problem of rigor in qualitative work revisited. *Advances in Nursing Science, 16*(2), 1-8.

Sandelowski, M. (1994). The proof is in the pottery: Toward a poetic for qualitative inquiry. In J. M. Morse (Ed.), *Critical issues in qualitative research methods.* Thousand Oaks, CA: Sage.

Sanjek, R. (Ed.). (1990). *Fieldnotes: The makings of anthropology.* Ithaca, NY: Cornell University Press

Sarnecky, M. T. (1990). Historiography: A legitimate research methodology for nursing. *Advances in Nursing Science, 12*(4), 1-10.

Sarnecky, M. T. (1993). Julia Catherine Stimson: Nurse and feminist. *Image, 25,* 113-119.

Schoenhofer, S. O. (1994). Transforming visions for nursing in the timeworld of Einstein's dreams. *Advances in Nursing Science, 16*(4), 1-8.

Schraeder, B. D. (1993). Assessment of measures to detect preschool academic risk in very-low-birth-weight children. *Nursing Research, 42,* 17-21.

Schultz, P. R., & Kerr, B. J. (1986). Comparative case study as a strategy for nursing research. In P. L. Chinn (Ed.), *Nursing research methodology.* Rockville, MD: Aspen.

Sheridan, A. (1980). *Michel Foucault: The will to truth.* London: Tavistock.

Siegel, S., & Castellan, N. J. (1988). *Nonparametric statistics for the behavioral sciences* (2nd ed.). New York: McGraw-Hill.

Simmons, H. (1992). Philosophic and scientific inquiry: The interface. In J. F. Kikuchi & H. Simmons (Eds.), *Philosophic inquiry in nursing.* Newbury Park, CA: Sage

Slakter, M. J., Wu, Y.-W. B., & Suzuki-Slakter, N. S. (1991). *, **, and ***; statistical nonsense at the . 00000 level. *Nursing Research, 40,* 248-249.

Smith, L. K., & Heshusius, L. (1986). Closing down the conversation: The end of the quantitative-qualitative debate among educational inquirers. *Educational Researcher, 15,* 4-12.

Smith, L. M. (1994). Biographical method. In N. K. Denzin & Y. S. Lincoln (Eds.), *Handbook of qualitative research.* Thousand Oaks, CA: Sage.

Smyth, K. A., & Yarandi, H. N. (1992). A path model of Type A and Type B responses to coping and stress in employed black women. *Nursing Research, 41,* 260-265.

Snyder-Halpern, R. (1994). An assessment taxonomy for designing nursing research programs. *Western Journal of Nursing Research, 16,* 81-93.

Sohier, R. (1993). Filial reconstruction: A theory of development through adversity. *Qualitative Health Research, 3,* 465-492.

Sparks, S. M. (1993). Electronic networking for nurses. *Image, 25,* 245-248.

Spiegelberg, H. (1982). *The phenomenological movement* (3rd ed.). The Hague, The Netherlands: Martinus Nijhoff.

Spradley, J. P. (1980). *Participant observation.* New York: Holt, Rinehart & Winston.

Staggers, N., & Mills, M. E. (1994). Nurse-computer interaction: Staff performance outcomes. *Nursing Research, 43,* 144-150.

Stapleton, T. J. (1983). *Husserl and Heidegger: The question of a phenomenological beginning.* Albany: State University of New York Press.

Stein, H. F. (1991). The role of some nonbiomedical parameters in clinical decision making: An ethnographic approach. *Qualitative Health Research, 1,* 6-26.

Stephenson, W. (1953). *The study of behavior.* Chicago: University of Chicago Press.

Stern, P. N. (1994). Eroding grounded theory. In J. M. Morse (Ed.), *Critical issues in qualitative research methods.* Thousand Oaks, CA: Sage.

Stevens, B. J. (1984). *Nursing theory: Analysis, application, evaluation* (2nd ed.). Boston: Little, Brown.

Stevens, P. E. (1989). A critical social reconceptualization of environment in nursing: Implications for methodology. *Advances in Nursing Science, 11*(2), 56-68.

Stevens, P. E. (1993). Marginalized women's access to health care: A feminist narrative analysis. *Advances in Nursing Science, 16*(2), 39-56.

Stevens, P. E. (1994). Protective strategies of lesbian clients in health care environments. *Research in Nursing and Health, 17,* 217-229.

Stevens, S. S. (1946). On the theory of scales of measurement. *Science, 103,* 677-680.

Stevens, S. Y. (1994). Aviation pioneers: World War II air evacuation nurses. *Nursing Research, 26,* 95-99.

Strauss, A. L., & Corbin, J. (1990). *Basics of qualitative research: Grounded theory procedures and techniques.* Newbury Park, CA: Sage.

Strauss, A. L., & Corbin, J. (1994). Grounded theory methodology: An overview. In N. K. Denzin & Y. S. Lincoln (Eds.), *Handbook of qualitative research.* Thousand Oaks, CA: Sage.

Strauss, A. L., & Glaser, B. G. (1975). *Chronic illness and the quality of life.* St. Louis: C. V. Mosby.

Street, A. F. (1992). *Inside nursing: A critical ethnography of clinical nursing practice.* Albany: State University of New York Press.

Stringer, M., & Librizzi, R. (1994). Complications following prenatal genetic procedures. *Nursing Research, 43,* 184-186.

Sudnow, D. (1967). *Passing on: The social organization of dying.* Englewood Cliffs, NJ: Prentice Hall.

Tanner, C. A., Benner, P., Chesla, C., & Gordon, D. R. (1993). The phenomenology of knowing the patient. *Image, 25,* 273-280.

Tappen, R. M. (1994). The effect of skill training on functional abilities of nursing home residents with dementia. *Research in Nursing and Health, 17,* 159-165.

Tesch, R. (1990). *Qualitative research: Analysis types and software tools.* New York: Falmer.

Thoits, P. (1982). Conceptual, methodological, and theoretical problems in studying social support as a buffer against life stress. *Journal of Health and Social Behavior, 23,* 145-159.

Thomas, J. (1993). *Doing critical ethnography.* Newbury Park, CA: Sage.

Thomas, R. M. (1984). Mapping meta-territory. *Educational Researcher, 13,* 16-18.

Thompson, J. B. (1982). *Paul Ricoeur: Hermeneutics and the human sciences.* New York: Cambridge University Press.

Thompson, J. L. (1991). Exploring gender and culture with Khmer refugee women: Reflections on participatory feminist research. *Advances in Nursing Science, 13*(3), 30-48.

Thorndike, E. L. (1918). The nature, purposes and general methods of measurements of educational products. In *The seventeenth yearbook of the National Society for the Study of Education* (Part 2). Bloomington, IL: Public School Publishing.

Thorne, S. (1994). Secondary analysis in qualitative research: Issues and implications. In J. M. Morse (Ed.), *Critical issues in qualitative research methods.* Thousand Oaks, CA: Sage.

Tripp-Reimer, T., Sorofman, B., Lauer, G., Martin, M., & Afifi, L. (1988). To be different from the world: Patterns of elder care among Iowa Old Order Amish. *Journal of Cross-Cultural Gerontology, 3,* 185-195.

Tukey, J. W. (1977). *Exploratory data analysis.* Reading, MA: Addison-Wesley.

Van Maanen, J. (1988). *Tales of the field: On writing ethnography.* Chicago: University of Chicago Press.

van Manen, M. (1986). *The tone of teaching.* Richmond Hill, Ontario: Scholastic-TAB.

van Manen, M. (1990). *Researching lived experience: Human science for an action sensitive pedagogy.* London, Ontario: University of Western Ontario & State University of New York Press.

Verran, J., & Ferketich, S. (1987a). Exploratory data analysis: Examining single distributions. *Western Journal of Nursing Research, 9,* 142-149.

Verran, J., & Ferketich, S. (1987b). Exploratory data analysis: Comparison of groups and variables. *Western Journal of Nursing Research, 9,* 617-625.

Wagner, T. J. (1985). Smoking behavior of nurses in western New York. *Nursing Research, 34,* 58-60.

Walker, B. L. (1993). Computer analysis of qualitative data: A comparison of three packages. *Qualitative Health Research, 3,* 91-111.

Walker, L. O., & Montgomery, E. (1994). Maternal identity and role attainment: Long-term relations to children's development. *Nursing Research, 43,* 105-110.

Waltz, C. F., Strickland, O. L., & Lenz, E. R. (1991). *Measurement in nursing research* (2nd ed.). Philadelphia: F. A. Davis.

Watson, J. (1985). *Nursing: Human science and human care: A theory of nursing.* Norwalk, CT: Appleton-Century-Crofts.

Webb, E. J., Campbell, D. T., Schwartz, R. B., Sechrest, L., & Grove, J. B. (1981). *Nonreactive measures in the social sciences* (2nd ed.). Boston: Houghton Mifflin.

Weiler, K. (1988). *Women teaching for change: Gender, class, and power.* Granby, MA: Bergin & Garvey.

Wells, S., Williamson, M., & Hooker, D. (1994). Fentanyl-induced chest wall rigidity in a neonate: A case report. *Heart and Lung, 23,* 196-198.

Wewers, M. E., & Lowe, N. K. (1990). A critical review of visual analogue scales in the measurement of clinical phenomena. *Research in Nursing and Health, 13,* 227-236.

White, J. H. (1991). Feminism, eating, and mental health. *Advances in Nursing Science, 13*(3), 68-80.

Whitney, J. D., Stotts, N. A., Goodson, W. H., & Janson-Bjerklie, S. (1993). The effects of activity and bed rest on tissue oxygen tension, perfusion, and plasma volume. *Nursing Research, 42,* 349-355.

Widerquist, J. G. (1992). The spirituality of Florence Nightingale. *Nursing Research, 41,* 49-55.

Wikoff, R. L., & Miller, P. (1991). Canonical analysis in nursing research. *Nursing Research, 40,* 367-370.

Wild, L. R. (1993). Caveat emptor: A critical analysis of the costs of drugs used for pain management. *Advances in Nursing Science, 16*(1), 52-61.

Williams, M. A., Oberst, M. T., & Bjorklund, B. C. (1994). Early outcomes after hip fracture among women discharged home and to nursing homes. *Research in Nursing and Health, 17,* 175-183.

Williamson, J. D., Karp, D. A., Dalphin, J. R., & Gray, P. S. (1982). *The research craft* (2nd ed.). Boston: Little, Brown.

Wilson, H. S., & Hutchinson, S. A. (1991). Triangulation of qualitative methods: Heideggerian hermeneutics and grounded theory, *Qualitative Health Research, 1,* 263-276.

Wilson, L. M., & Fitzpatrick, J. J. (1984). Dialectical thinking as a means of understanding systems-in-development: Relevance to Rogers's principles. *Advances in Nursing Science, 6*(2), 24-41.

Workman, M. L., & Livingston, G. K. (1993). Testing the sensitivity of a biologic assay for mutagenicity. *Nursing Research, 42,* 373-375.

Yarandi, H. N. (1993). Coding dummy variables and calculating the relative risk in a logistic regression. *Nursing Research, 42,* 312-314.

Yarandi, H. N., & Simpson, S. H. (1991). The logistic regression model and the odds of testing HIV positive. *Nursing Research, 40,* 372-373.

Yin, R. K. (1989). *Case study research: Design and methods* (2nd ed.). Beverly Hills, CA: Sage.

Yow, V. R. (1994). *Recording oral history: A practical guide for social scientists.* Thousand Oaks, CA: Sage.

Zachariah, R. (1994). Maternal-fetal attachment: Influence of mother-daughter and husband-wife relationships. *Research in Nursing and Health, 17,* 37-44.

Zielstorff, R. D., Hudgings, C. I., Grobe, S. J., & the National Commission on Nursing Implementation Project (NCNIP) Task Force on Nursing Information Systems. (1993). *Next-generation nursing information systems: Essential characteristics for professional practice.* Washington, DC: American Nurses Association.

ABOUT THE AUTHORS

BETHEL ANN POWERS is Associate Professor of Nursing at the University of Rochester, where she received a master of science degree in nursing (1971) and a Ph.D. in anthropology (1980). Her clinical research interests are in gerontological nursing, and she has published articles in nursing and interdisciplinary journals about her study of social networks of elderly institutionalized people. She has taught classes on nursing theory and research to baccalaureate, master's, and doctoral students in nursing, and she developed a qualitative research course for doctoral students in the School of Nursing. She also reviews manuscripts for *Image* and *Research in Nursing & Health*.

THOMAS R. KNAPP (Ed.D., Harvard, 1959) is Professor of Nursing and Education at The Ohio State University. His specialty is research methodology (statistics, measurement, research design). He has published several articles on validity and reliability and other methodological topics, and has contributed to the research literature in demography, economics, education, nursing, and psychology. He also serves as a referee for several research journals, including *Psychological Bulletin* and *Research in Nursing & Health*.